I0837443

CBD Oil ~

Fact vs Fiction:

Finding truth among all the lies.

CBD… CBC, CBG, CBL, CBN, CBT, and many other cannabinoids

Real Science, Honest Legalities, Common Sense Applications

© Terry Mercer, 2018,2019

The Science, Safe Use, the Difference between the Real Stuff vs Fake Stuff, Spotting the Difference in Marketing Hype and Truth, Some Reality in the Legalities, and a Brief Interesting History of Cannabis – how it got here, and where things are really going… are all discussed within the following pages.

ISBN: 9781793897336

Who will benefit from this book?

> ➤ People that want to learn some truths, reality, actual science, and real legal issues… from someone that is not trying to sell them any miracle or magical product.

> ➤ It can help those wanting to learn how to wade through the hyperbole… learn how to protect yourself better… potentially even from scammers and some legally regarding insurance, job, and the system in general.

> ➤ It will answer many questions, some you didn't know you had… and can help optimize whatever you are doing (especially if you have chronic issues or medical issue).

> ➤ People that are not already smoking, eating, or otherwise using cannabis, or derived products, in some fashion.

> ➤ Learn what you really are (and aren't) risking in, even with the recent 'decriminalization' of 'hemp' and industrial hemp derived products.

Finding some real answers, despite the marketing hype and media's bias, and the outright misinformation from those MLM's and network marketers, and home sales people. Getting to the truth – one way or the other. Science really does matter, and honestly exists for many things.

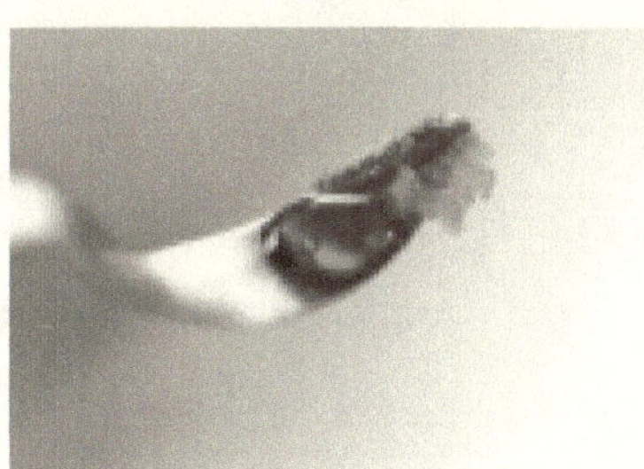
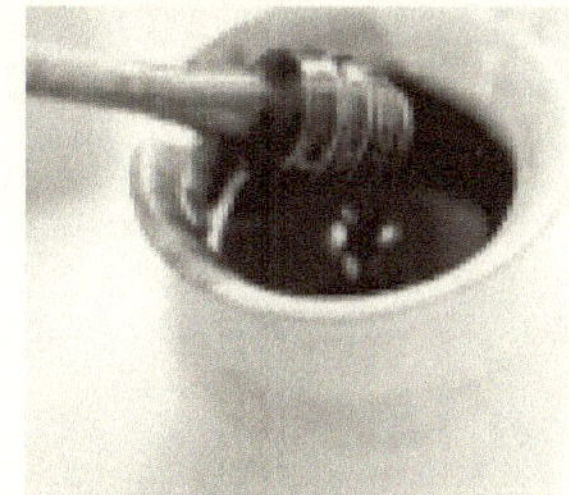

PREFACE

We do NOT have, sell, represent, promote, or profit from any CBD manufacturer, CBD product, THC supplier, or cannabis industry person, product, or company.

We bothered gathering and sorting through all the information we could, hopeful to get some real and honest answers, because WE HAVE family, friends, and clients that suffer from debilitating and unpredictable seizures, some have since birth; and friends with Parkinson's. Many suffer with long term chronic pain that surgery and blockers have not helped.

Like most people over the last fifty years, we have lost dozens of loved ones to Cancer; and know many that are actively battling it today. **We took this project seriously, and actively pay closer attention when rumors circulate, especially in the scientific community, about any nutrient, supplement, or drugs that *might* help those suffering. The information, studies, and links contained herein became a particular interest, and hope they can help you!**

We waded through a few thousand scientific abstracts, articles, and laws. Asked some key questions to people educated on the topics, which study and deal with the subjects on a regular basis. Our goal was to gather and evaluate information, as honestly, ethically, and rationally as possible, with the most hope and least bias, seeking solutions and answers... employing common sense, and a sense of reality.

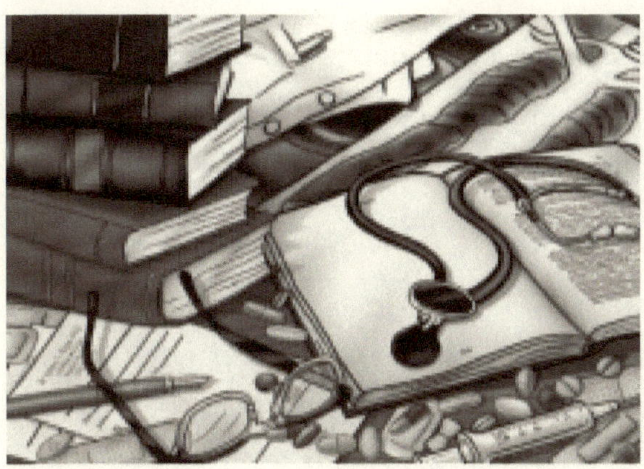

Personally, I have been active in the Health Industry, for people and animals, primarily dealing with joints and digestion, with some regarding critical care meals, reproduction supplements, and general health primarily for MD's Choice, Inc. since 1995. Armed with my meniscal degree in Physical Sciences from the 80's, a pile of common sense, rational logic, an ethical desire to find some truth, and nearly twenty years of working directly with the doctors & nutritionists.

Over the years, I have edited thousands of pages for doctors I have been working with. I also helped design and maintain dozens of health related websites, hundreds of product labels, and assorted marketing materials over the last twenty plus years. Ultimately, in the Health Industry, I am just a well-trained parrot, with a clear understanding of my own limitations, and foundation of experience.

I am not a doctor or nutritionist, though I have worked closely with a variety of them for over twenty years. I am a problem solver, and educationally focused citizen that can both wade through scientific research and has some smart friends.

Understand, each body and case is different. Their diet, exercise routine, genetics, other medications & treatments, medical history, environment, must all be considered. What works for one might not work well, or the same, for another.

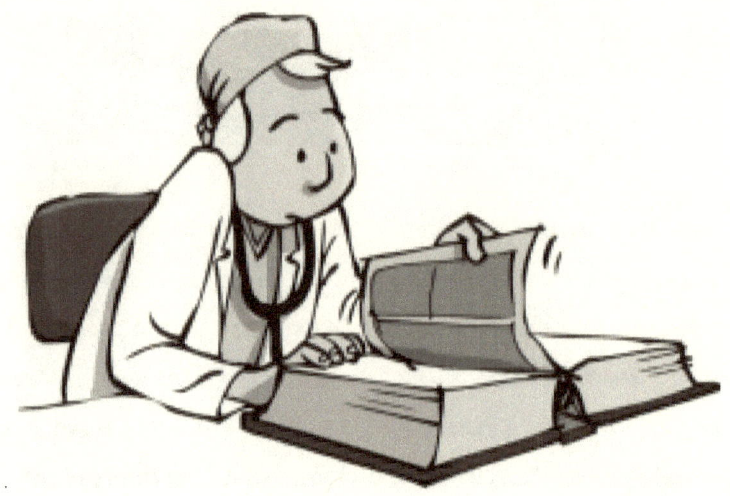

Biology and physiology in mammals have some absolute similarities, and generalities, as the vast majority of bodies function in the same way. They respond to the right forms of vitamins, minerals, trace minerals, amino acids, enzymes, and certain nutrients in very similar fashions, for specific and certain issues.

However, human bodies tend to respond to drugs with more variability, because our environments, diet, exercise, and daily intake is so vastly different. (Most animals 'eat' and 'do' essentially the same thing in a given geographical region, not true with humans). Whether pharmaceutical or natural, there are often more differences and side effects with 'drugs' (including plant derived drugs), depending on what ALL a body is doing, taking, or using... amount, frequency, and longevity.

According to the studies, cannabis seems to be a safe alternative for many types of drugs, serving a variety of purposes, with few exceptions focused on SYMPTOMS. Never a report of an over-dose from actual marijuana, or real CBD Oil, causing a death. Proof that some valid treatments, for some specific types of medical issues, have been shown to exist from either THC or CBD, often BOTH in some ratio in the treatment protocol.

It was suggested that we share some of what we've learned over the years, so other's might benefit, and have more information on the topic to think about, maybe saving them valuable time, helping them find a path, and likely learn something more in the process; so they would have more to discuss with their doctor, or professional healthcare provider, as necessary.

NOTHING HEREIN has been approved by the FDA, or any other government agency. The information contained herein is not intended to give any medical advice, or to prevent, treat, or cure any ailment or disease. Nor any legal advice.

"Learning without thinking is useless. Thinking without learning is dangerous." ~ Confucius

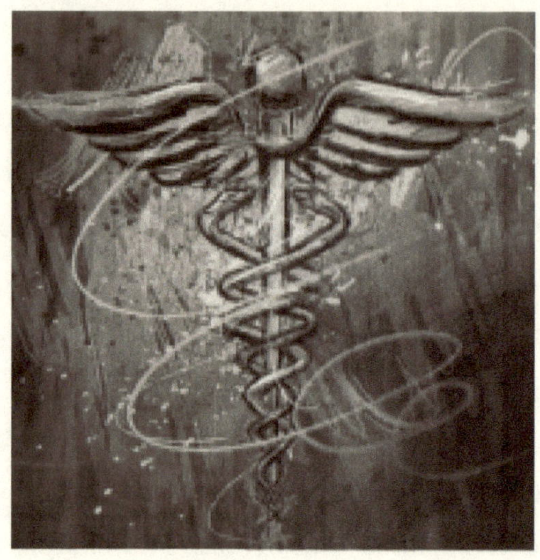

Use this information at your own risk, and PLEASE consult a specialist in the field you (or your loved one) has a problem with, whether medical or legal, person or pet. Do not blindly believe anyone – person or company - selling bottles of CBD Oil (hemp or cannabis based products) at the swap meets, Flea Markets, on-line, or in books without learning to ask the right questions, and request the right documentation. Above all, considering all sides, and the reality of what it can do, absolutely cannot do, and ALL the real potential costs!

Everyone wants hope, especially when they are sick, in pain, or diagnosed with some nasty disease that does not seem to have any cure or effective treatment that is not riddled with a pile of side effects. Most people would like a quick fix, or magic potion that cures disease, improves health, and increases longevity. At nearly 60 years old, believe me when I say I would love all those things too. **Look at the SCIENCE; consider the relevance, reality, and significance to your needs.**

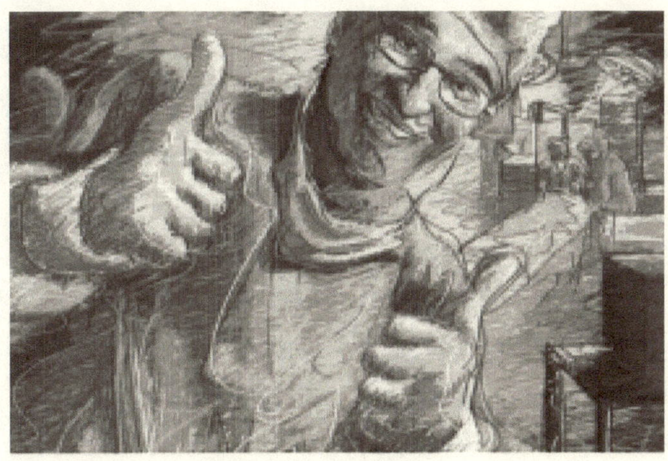

Specialists spend 10 to 16 years just getting their degree in that specialty, their residency and internships, before forming a foundation to their professional opinion with some actual cases and experience under their belt. Add-in their yearly 'continuing education,' just to maintain their license, which is required (at least here in the United States), all the specialized tools used in their examinations, and you can see why most of those professionals are apprised of the latest approved treatments, procedures, breaking peer reviewed studies, and usually have the best answers for any disease or issue they specialized in.

That being said, the average surgeon and specialist only has to take a semester or two of NUTRITION (unless they opted for more, or it's otherwise required because of their specialty or choice).

It should be understood that 'they' are all human, and no single person or team, is absolutely perfect, or knows everything, all the time. The broader the training – education and experience – of the team, often the better their diagnosis, treatment protocols, suggested solutions, and success rates.

Some professionals are more oriented toward surgery, some toward prevention (diet, nutrition, and exercise), and some toward aggressive treatment (drugs, chemicals, or specialty treatments), while other's just focus on reducing the pain and suffering.

You need to determine what type of doctor best suits your needs. However, their extensive training, particularly when they specialized in the problem you're having, along with their ability to SEE and TOUCH the patient, RUN the tests, and evaluate the individual situation, gives them an incredible unique advantage you should never just ignore.

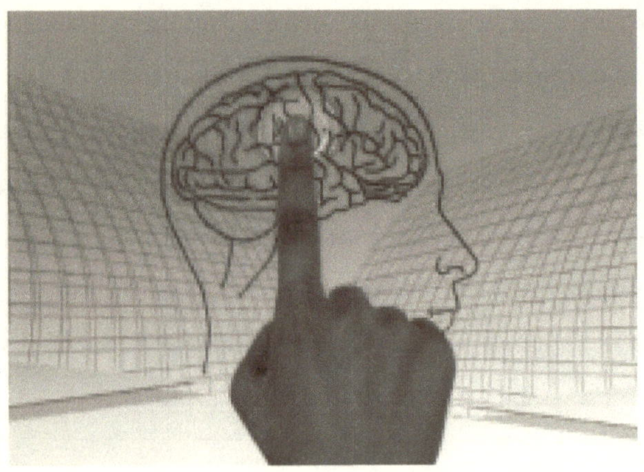

If you do not like or trust them, get a second opinion… from another professional.

Do not rely upon 'Dr. Google,' or solely on some stranger on line (or even in a book). I frankly do not care what their credentials are, UNLESS THEY EXAMINE YOU, AND KNOW YOUR CASE, they can only speak, write, or discuss generalities. Not specifics to YOU, and your health concerns!

A proper diagnosis relies on test results, hands on observation with direct response to questions, and an examination. NOT a 'Google Search' or any book!

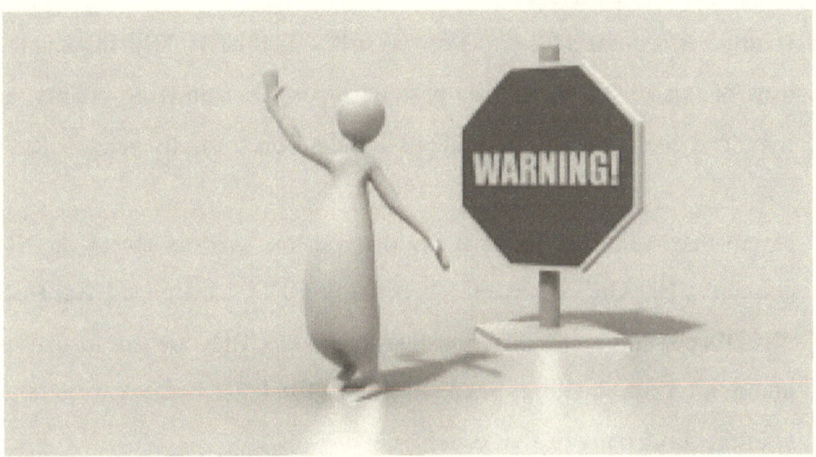

Consult YOUR DOCTOR before using any cannabis product(s), and honestly consider the potential legal ramifications, and actual liability potential, which really could be a double edge sword… even in 'legal' states.

Understand, there is a massive difference between true 'cannabis' CBD oil, and the generic 'industrial hemp' seed oil that is cropping up everywhere with piles of false claims attached to them! Throughout this book, I will explain the differences… the science, legalities, as well as what to look for, if you are truly looking for 'the good stuff.'

The reality is that some claims marketers make are based in some truth, but the greater reality is that most science has absolutely nothing to do with the product they are pushing or promoting. And many of the claims are absolutely not true (of any CBD oil based product), like those claiming Arthritis can be cured (not true, but pain *might* be reduced for some people… as the underlying problem gets worse).

It truly has become a **Caveat Emptor = BUYER BEWARE** market, with tons of 'snake oil' type dishonest sales-people, marketing claims, and hype that doesn't really fit or apply to the product usually being sold.

Hemp Seed Oil sold in most health food and grocery stores do NOT contain 'CBD Oil' or have the benefits of CBD. Understand that Hemp SEED's contain many different nutrients, but CBDs are not in that list, and don't exist in Hemp Seed Oil unless the CBD isolates were added after the processing of the seeds!

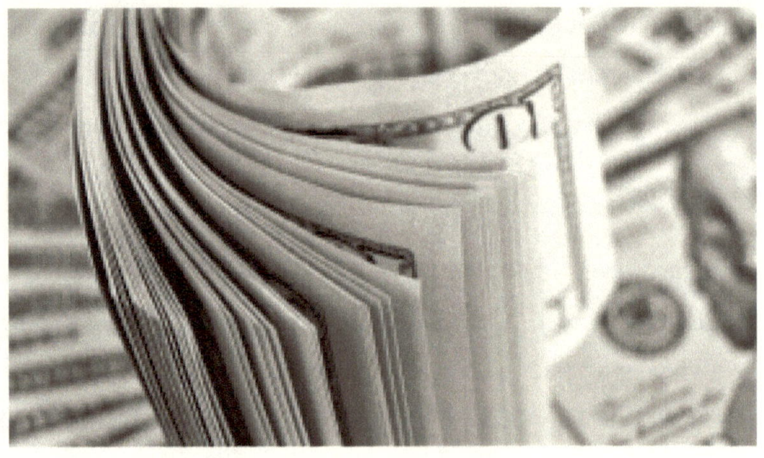

**There are also potential legal concerns,
which are discussed later in this book.**

Page Intentionally Left Blank for Your Own Notes:

DECEMBER 20TH, 2018 UPDATE

The 2018 farm bill or 'Agriculture Improvement Act of 2018' is United States legislation, which passed, and has been signed into law on this date, which reauthorizes and updates many expenditures in the prior US farm bill, 'the Agricultural Act of 2014.'

In a statement following Thursday's bill signing in Washington, Scott Gottlieb, the FDA Commissioner, restated his agency's stance that CBD, even after the Farm Bill was signed: "IS CONSIDERED A DRUG, if sold as an ingredient to prevent, treat, or cure any disease or medical condition, and therefore illegal to add to food or health products without approval from this agency. Selling unapproved products with unsubstantiated therapeutic claims is not only a violation of the law, but also can put patients at risk, as these products have not been proven to be safe or effective."

The 2018 bill has an estimated cost of at least $867 billion US Dollars in the reconciled farm bill. It was passed by the Senate (87 Yeas to just 13 Nays) on December 11, 2018, and by the House on December 12 (369 Yeas vs 47 Nays); so very bi-partisan. Then, on December 20th, 2018 it received President Trump's signature and became the current law.

The bill "largely continues current farm and nutrition policies," and does not include any of the proposed new requirements for SNAP (food stamps) recipients that existed in earlier drafts of this same bill earlier in the year.

Just to be clear, **HR2(115) is now law, but ONLY UNTIL 2023**, where congress may decide to change things again. This bill (commonly known as the 'Farm Bill') reauthorizes through FY2023 (Fiscal Year) and modifies

Department of Agriculture (USDA) programs that address:

- commodity support,

- conservation,

- trade and international food aid,

- nutrition assistance,

- farm credit,

- rural development,

- research and extension activities,

- forestry,

- energy,

- horticulture, and

- crop insurance.

The bill modifies agriculture and nutrition policies to:

- require farmers to make a new election to obtain either Price Loss Coverage or Agricultural Risk Coverage for the 2019-2023 crop years, which may be changed for the 2021-2023 crop years;

- replace the Dairy Margin Protection Program with Dairy Risk Coverage and modify coverage levels and premiums;

- reduce the adjusted gross income limitation for receiving benefits under commodity and conservation programs;

- modify funding levels and requirements for several conservation programs,

- consolidate several existing trade and export promotion programs into a new Priority Trade Promotion, Development, and Assistance program;

- establish an interstate data system to prevent the simultaneous issuance of Supplemental Nutrition Assistance Program (SNAP, formerly known as the food stamp program) benefits to an individual by more than one state;

- increase the loan limits for farm ownership and operating loans;
- modify the experience requirement for farm ownership loans;
- authorize a categorical exclusion from requirements for environmental assessments and environmental impact statements for certain forest management projects with the primary purpose of protecting, restoring, or improving habitat for the greater sage-grouse or mule deer; and
- make Indian tribes and tribal organizations eligible for supplemental agricultural disaster assistance programs;
- modify the organic certification requirements for imported agricultural products.

And lastly, and why it's important to this topic:

- legalize industrial hemp and make hemp producers eligible for the federal crop insurance program;

Again, this 2018 Farm Bill, signed into law on December 20th, 2018, decriminalizes **INDUSTRIAL** HEMP federally. This is a type of cannabis, not 'pot' (or marijuana). It is the form of with lower **THC levels (3% or less), than the levels found in 'marijuana.'** This law specifically removed Industrial Hemp and CBD Oil derived from such hemp from the FEDERAL SCHEDULES, as a Controlled Substance, **which will drastically change the market, and potentially clarifies many of the laws in this nation.**

Analysts have projected that this one change alone will allow the hemp industry, which is currently doing about $2 Billion a year in sales, to skyrocket into an industry doing more than $23 billion a year by 2022. That should have a significant impact on jobs, unemployment, and future investments. REMEMBER, the same type of thing happened under President Carter... but he decriminalized ALL CANNABIS, for a time... but it was reinstated just a couple years later when President Reagan upped the anti on the War on Drugs President Nixon stated in 1972.

The 'Farm Bill' is voted on, AND CHANGED, about every 4 to 8 years... or basically once every newly elected President. However, if the positive medical studies continue piling up, the safety remains (i.e., no overdoses or deaths), and the money is really producing jobs… it's likely **Industrial Hemp and CBD oils with low THC will never become a 'Scheduled Drug' in America again in our lifetime.** However, it continue to be regulated, just like ANY HERBAL SUPPLEMTENT, and ingredient(s), intended to help prevent, heal, treat, cure, or otherwise effect any disease. The Farm Bill, and non-specific verbiage, gives an implied approval, which is why the FDA jumped out there so quickly to remind people what the laws really are, and who are impacted, and why. The FDA has said that there are three ingredients derived from industrial hemp — hulled hemp seeds, hemp seed protein and hemp seed oil — which are deemed GRAS (generally regarded as safe) and are approved for to be sold "AS FOODSTUFF" without additional approvals, as long as marketers do not make claims that those products can prevent, treat, or cure any disease.

The Farm Bill is absolutely a start, but ultimately opens the door for scammers, manipulators, and piles of false claims. There are also potential legal concerns, which are discussed later in this book.

Page Intentionally Left Blank for Your Own Notes:

What is CBD Oil?

CBD stands for 'cannabidiol.' Pronounced can-nab-id-all.

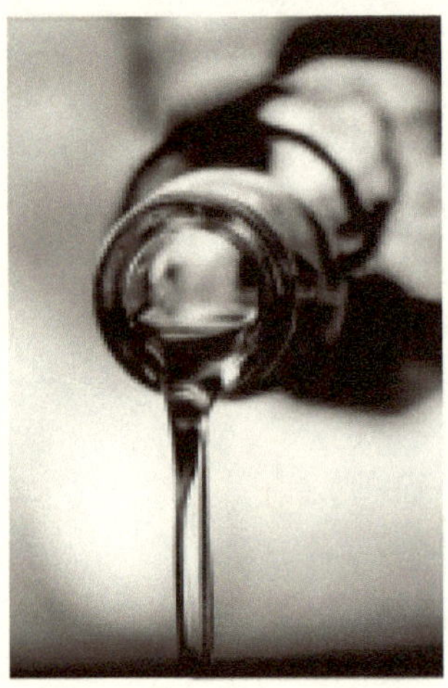

It is just one of nearly 500 cannabinoids that are naturally occurring chemicals found in cannabis plants. Cannabinoids, themselves, are not psychotropic (they won't get someone 'high'), and do not have any 'nutritional value.' CBD is just one of over one hundred cannabinoids that exist in cannabis plants, which have been officially named, and are studied the most often by research scientists.

CBD oil can be consistently extracted from the stalk & leaves (also buds and flowers, which contain higher levels of THC). Seeds are said to have NO CBD's. Much like the juice from grapes, THC and CBD are components of all species of cannabis plants, just different levels of the key chemicals unique to that species… depending on the strain, where the raw material is from, and the manufacturing process. THC is absolutely a component of the cannabis plant, though it is fractional (usually 0.3% or less, in the 'Industrial Hemp'); however, the differences go beyond just differences potency, color, or taste; but the levels of all the OTHER components also.

Cannabis seeds contain about 30% OIL by weight, and there is absolutely NO CBD in the oil produced from hemp seeds. So if anyone tells you (or says on their label or marketing material) that seeds are the 'source' of their CBD oils, especially if the word 'HEMP' is used anywhere in junction with that product, you should question everything they claim! The source, the science, and the other ingredients that company employed in manufacturing their product. Note: seeds from marijuana contain higher levels of THC, while Industrial Hemp seed have just a fraction of a percent (of THC).

Fiber from hemp is also NOT the optimal source for CBD, despite marketing claims. Most of those assertions are being made when the Industrial Hemp was deemed accepted in some states, and was not being as actively pursued by the DEA. Hemp contains far less cannabidiol CBD (quantity, and potency) per pound, than most any of the CBD-rich cannabis strains leaves and flower tops (of marijuana).

So, all that marketing hype claiming they are avoiding THC by using industrial hemp, is also restricting the concentration and potency of the CBD oils, which have most of the medicinal benefits (and scientific support, abstracts, and research). The studies referenced, proof of some medicinal benefits, are the only reason most people are even consider the use of CBD products (hoping to stay legal). In the legal states, people are usually just going to a dispensary and getting a CBD made from actual marijuana, with low THC (but higher than 0.3%).

If you think of cannabis like grapes, it might make a little more sense. Grapes can be grape juice, raisins, vinegar, jam, jelly, butter, marmalade, or when fermented, they can be cheap to fine wine, brandy, or even expensive Champagne… and a variety of other products. The reality is that each are different, and the same logic is true with most cannabis products. The varieties and strains are all different! With different levels of the key ingredients, different production processes, different harvesting methods, and different additives.

Understand, unless CBD's are being added to their hemp seed extract, they might not actually have any of the sought after medicinal cannabidiols in their product. Since there is currently no requirements that label claims have to be true or honest, it is truly all about the integrity of the company, and the certificate of analysis (COA). **If hemp seed oil extract is the base, used as the diluent or to reduce the potency of the CBD oils, then a COA is even more important,** to insure what is actually in the product, and what isn't.

In addition, the actual levels and types of cannabinoids are subject to change from manufacturer to manufacturer, strain to strain, and even harvest to harvest. Remember there are over 500 identified cannabinoids, but just 113 that have been officially named in cannabis plants; and CBD is just one of those 500… which has the second most science behind it, behind only THC.

While hemp seed oil has nutritional value, because it contains a lot of omega 3 & 6 polyunsaturated fatty acids (without the fish oil smell or after taste), there are also trace amounts of calcium, iron, magnesium, phosphorus, potassium, sodium, sulfur, zinc, vitamin E, and even protein in hemp oil. It is NOT psychoactive, containing less than .03% THC, but does NOT contain CBD oil, or any other cannabinoids, **unless they are added after the pressing.**

Anyone that tells you 'hemp seed oil' contains CBD, without it being specifically added to, is greatly misinformed and probably isn't really testing their product… because there aren't CBD's in hemp seeds.

In general, 'hemp' is referring to 'industrial hemp,' whereas 'cannabis oil' is from non-industrial hemp. There is also product made with 'hemp seed,' which has zero CBD's, unless added after the pressing. Pure unrefined cannabis oil is dark green in color. All the nutrition is preserved when it is cold pressed (no heat or solvents). Huge amounts of industrial hemp leaves and flowers are required to get a small amount of CBD, which necessarily increases the risks of contaminants.

Cannabis is a 'bio-accumulator' that naturally and normally draws toxins from the soil as it grows. It is one of the most cost-effective methods of cleaning the environment of toxic heavy metals and organic pollutants. It is also the danger, and concern, when not grown in food-grade conditions, and safe soils.

The cheap stuff is often sold, with false marketing or label claims. Those claims that might be perfectly true for the 'right type' and 'good' product, but has absolutely nothing to do with what they are selling. Hemp oils, and cannabis oils, **grown in non-food grade soils have been found to be high in lead, mercury, and other heavy metals that accumulate in the body.**

Those foreign manufactured products, and less than responsible, companies pushing CBD oils with less than responsible and ethical standards, either growing in bad soils or adding synthetics or other herbs, are causing distrust, and hurting the future of the industry. The easiest way to solve that problem would be independent third party testing AFTER BOTTLING – for CBD level, THC levels, all common toxins, microbials, pesticides, herbicides, and other cannabinoids in the plant.

Industrial hemp is not cultivated to produce buds, and therefore lacks the potency of the primary component (THC) that forms the marijuana high. With Marijuana, the highest concentration of THC is formed in resin glands on the buds and flowers of the female plants. There is far less in the male plants, and even less in the Industrial Hemp plants. Despite some advertising and marketing claims, Cannabis Oil is absolutely different than Hemp Oil… even more different than raisins to wine, although made from the same species of plants.

Today, mostly because of the videos of young children with drug resistant epilepsy, having an average of 300 seizures a day, so dramatically and positively responding to CBD Oils… dropping to fewer than 20 a day, most with less intensity and duration, people around the world took notice. The video was viewed hundreds of millions of times. It reignited the discussions and push for scientific studies and legalization; but then accelerated it, with a public outcry of truth and justice, because the family had to move, to keep CPS (Children's Protective Services) from trying to take their child from them, for giving her a 'schedule 1 controlled substance.'

Citizens rallied, demanding more actual scientific studies; which have been happening these last few years. Discussions of choice, and legalized medical use of cannabis were pushed to the forefront. States started jumping on the legalization bandwagon; mostly because of the PROFIT THEY SEE NOW. For many states, the cannabis industry (Marijuana, CBD) are viewed as the casinos and lottery were in the 90's…just another income stream. The difference is cannabis actually has some actual benefit, and is far less addicting.

How and why it helps is important. What it does (and does not do) in the body is also important. Science is proving, and disproving, many of the rumors, claims, and learning new stuff every year, with dozens of new studies from around the world. There has been significantly more good science the last couple decades.

History and science prove Cannabis has actually been used, around the world, for medicinal purposes, for thousands of years. (More about all that in the history section, for those interested).

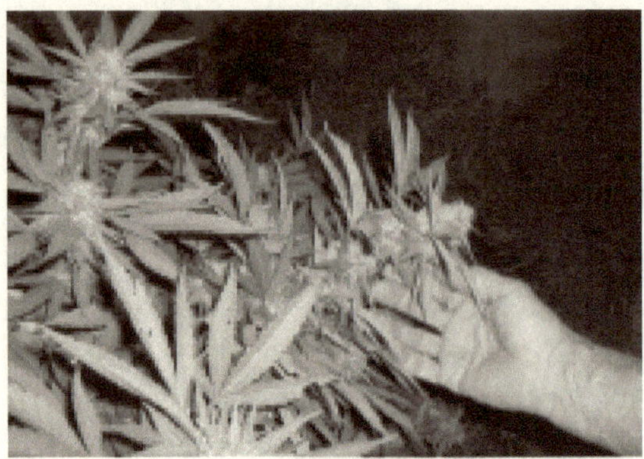

In reality, just like the prohibition on alcohol, the use of cannabis will continue, whether it is legal or not. **Cannabis is here, has been for centuries, and will be as long as there are humans walking this planet.**

The questions that should be asked are:
- WHAT IS SAFE?
- What is really legal?
- What is real? And,
- How might it help or hurt you, or you loved one?

CBD is the second most popular, and most studied, component of the cannabis plant that is regularly discussed, right behind THC. These two components are probably the most commonly discussed chemicals in herbs over the last sixty years.

CBD can effectively be manufactured from either marijuana or hemp, both of which are cannabis. That last fact is a large part of the problem, and why it has not been readily legalized at the federal level, in all states, or even in all other countries.

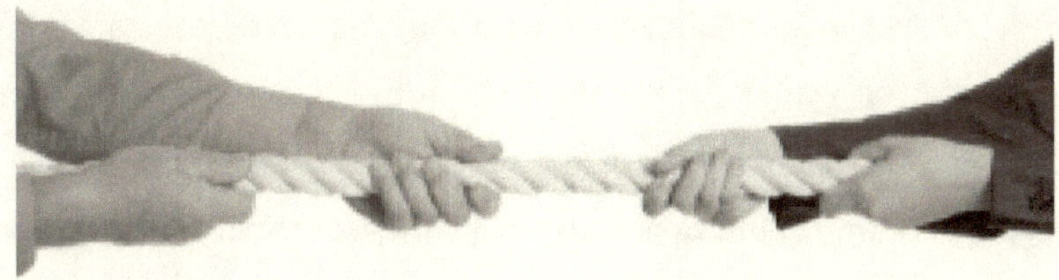

There is an absolute difference between **UNENFORCED LAWS** and **LEGAL**. Today, most government officials are overlooking, ignoring, and avoiding CBD Oils, because of the Ninth Circuit Court ruling a couple years ago. **That did not legalize it**, but instead slammed things into a grey area; creating a 'loop hole,' which the federal government has officially, at least for now, decided not to enforce much (or often). Again, different from 'not at all.' The 2018 Farm Bill pushed things forward; but ultimately dumped things directly into the lap of the FDA over claims (and the DEA if the levels of THC are higher than .03%).

In general, the high-quality CBD products with low THC contain less than 0.3% THC are manufactured from the leaves and stalks of industrial hemp (not the seeds, buds, or flowers). If they truly have less than 0.3% THC, there are **people that will tell you they are legal in all 50 states, and that is misinformation is all over the internet**, with absolute false claims. Which potentially, and partially, changed on December 20th, 2018, when President Trump signed the Farm Bill, and removed Industrial Hemp, and derivatives from it, from the Controlled Substance Schedules… FEDERALLY!

Previously, if you are in a legal state, the state officials weren't likely to come after you, or your property. In the non-legal states, the federal government was also unlikely to come after you, unless the state officials request it, or you're deemed to be a part of some interstate criminal operation, or you've ticked off the wrong person(s) in power. Today, and since 2017, low quantities of marijuana is often considered like a speeding ticket or minor offense, even in most illegal states (with a few exceptions… to remind people of the actual laws).

Under federal law, ANYTHING and EVERYTHING made from, or a component of, the cannabis sativa, the 'marijuana' or NON-Industrial form of the cannabis plants, not specifically approved by the federal government is STILL 100% against federal laws, and STILL listed as a Schedule 1 Controlled Substance. That is the legal reality.

Rusty Payne, with the US DEA, recently said, "The law on the subject is very clear. It is not legal. It's just not." However, according to him, , neither the DEA nor DOJ are actively or aggressively pursuing arrests or convictions related to marijuana, CBD, or other cannabis related products at this time. He listed three reasons: a) cannabis has not killed anyone, b) our nation is battling an opioid epidemic, which is killing people, and deserves more of their time and focus, and c) there really is some promising science regarding medical use of cannabis products for certain health issues.

So, according to Mr. Payne, the federal enforcement will be little to nothing, unless ordered otherwise, although it really is federally illegal, until laws change. However, the reality that it is still against the law has enabled some law enforcement officers, for some agency, usually DEA or FBI, or even the local police, to come in and physically confiscate property, and even arrest people over just CBD Oil, gummy bears, or pot. Threatening them with serious drug charges, fines, and lengthy prison sentences.

The DEA firmly believes the Farm Bill permits CBD research only — not CBD marketing and sales to the general public, or use by unauthorized people (or pets). Quite the conundrum, huh?

CBD Oil is currently being pushed and hyped, especially here in America, in everything from epilepsy treatments, to muscle rubs, claims of cancer cures, pain relievers, and virtually everything else... including pet-calming drops. It is important to understand the very real difference between 'drugs' and 'supplements.' The FDA will smack down any company they catch making drug claims without specific science, and actual studies that can be confirmed by third parties, and repeated... and is USING THE SAME PRODUCT FORMULA the claims are on. HUGE difference from 'it's all the same' - because the reality is that it is not.

It is manufactured in nearly every conceivable form, but regardless of form, quality, safety, or actual science should be considered. The reality is that there is some real good science and a lot of promise on the 'good stuff' –**There is a lot of fake, and drastically cut, and questionable stuff out there in the market place**. Some that is really not made from or with cannabis, some with truly low THC content <0.3%, some with unknown amounts that do not match label claims; as well as some with levels high enough you could test positive for THC.

Quality, caution, consistency, potency, and science are important, if you are trying to treat something.

You can hand a recipe to 10 different people for an apple pie, and when they fix their pies, you'll get 10 different looking pies, each with subtly different tastes, and even slightly different actual nutrients, flavors, and even potentially different smells, and nutrient levels.

The cheap Hemp Oils do NOT contain therapeutic levels of CBD oil, and will not produce the results any of the medical studies have discussed or tested for. Hemp Oil is NOT the same as quality, potency, or concentration of real 'Cannabis Oil' which contains all the necessary cannabinoids (CBD being just one of over 500). Hemp oil can have nutritional value, and benefits, just not therapeutic CBD benefits.

Page Intentionally Left Blank for Your Own Notes:

WHAT CBD DOES (& DOESN'T DO):

cGMP (certified Good Manufacturing Practices) doesn't necessarily mean the same in the cannabis world that it does with the rest of the nutritional supplements, or even conventional herbal remedies. At this point, the cGMP logo or claim might not be the best way to determine if a product is real, or their label is accurate. It can really only tell you that the bottling plant is considered 'generally clean and safe.'

Claims that a product is manufactured in a "FDA Inspected" facility is meaningless, though it does usually mean it's not made in someone's bathtub or home kitchen with pets and kids running around. The FDA might 'inspect' a facility making OTHER GOODS, but it does not inspect or oversee the manufacturing of non-FDA approved cannabis goods, in any facility; as it is AGAINST FEDERAL LAW!

The claims surrounding CBD and cannabis products are vast, and some actual science is absolutely worth following; some are complete lies. It really does seem to actually help with many common medial problems, and has for centuries. Check out the list below, to see what has proven effective, and how; as well as what hasn't.

EPILEPSY - Like lessening both the intensity and frequency of some forms of epileptic seizures, especially repetitive drug resistant debilitating seizures. Understand, while CBD Oil has a growing amount lot of science, and some significant proof in helping quell certain types of seizures – frequency and/or severity, understand that science does not affect all types, or work for all people.

Buried in vintage medical books, a paper was found, from 1843, when a British doctor named William O'Shaughnessy published his article detailing how cannabis oil had arrested an infant's relentless convulsions.

1980 STUDY IN PHARMACOLOGY was one of the very first studies published regarding CBD Oil. They published their findings conducted on eight volunteers, during a study in which they tested 15 patients with epilepsy and chronic seizures (23 total people). The goal was to determine safety, specifically looking for any side effects of CBD Oil when consumed daily, at high doses, for a month. Their reported conclusions were, 'All patients AND the volunteers tolerated CBD very well and no signs of toxicity or serious side effects were detected on examination.'

2014 PEDIATRIC STUDY INVOLVING CBD OIL AT "CHILDREN'S OF ALABAMA", was officially authorized by the Alabama State legislature in 2014, after millions of people saw the dramatic video of a child suffering from multiple intractable grand maul seizures each day, which were significantly quieted by just a few drops of CBD Oil a few times a day. It truly was amazing. The legislation allowing the testing and use for epileptics, known as 'Carly's Law' passed without much delay or debate. Help, at least for some, appeared to be on the way...

with many scientists jumping on board filing for funds necessary to conduct a variety of studies for their medical specialty. They wanted to officially be on record, as part of the proof or disproof, of the effects. Parents, and doctors, were signing up kids with this problem right and left, some even moving from out of state, in hopes of finding a cure for their child.

2015, SOOTHING SEIZURES ANOTHER STUDY ABOUT CBD OIL caught our eye, it was still 'in process.' The claims are miraculous, and were being reported in official journals by 2016. The implications and promise started getting pushed and promoted heavily by the main stream media throughout the 2016 elections. More states approved the use of 'medical marijuana' and a couple more jumped on the 'recreational use' bandwagon (with limits and, of course, taxation). There became much more talk about pushing for some federal legalization to remove the 'Schedule 1' listing on Marijuana altogether, especially from CBD Oil used for medical purposes.

In another important case, parents described severe seizures in their six months old daughter. They started in started in May 2013. Infantile spasms, are what the doctors called them. The parents described what they saw, a startle reflex—her arms rigid at her side, her face a frozen mask of fear, her eyes fluttering from side to side. Their daughter, Addelyn Patrick's little brain raced and surged, as though an electromagnetic storm were sweeping through her. "It's your worst possible nightmare," her mother, Meagan, says. "Just awful, awful, awful to watch your child in pain, in fear, and there's nothing you can do to stop it." By early 2016 the Patrick's had made up their minds. They would move to Colorado to join the movement. "It was a no-brainer," Meagan says. "If they were growing something on Mars that might help Addy, I'd be in my backyard building a spaceship."

2017 PROVIG TREATMET OF EPILEPSY, though limited to certain forms, the results were piling up according to the media. GW Pharmaceuticals, known as Greenwich Biosciences in the U.S., completed its new drug application for Epidiolex, which is a formulation of CBD to treat seizures. If it gets full unrestricted approved, Epidiolex could easily earn over $2.2 billion a year by 2025, according to analysts at Goldman Sachs. The initial study results were released, showing that out of 51 test subjects, 50% saw sustained significantly improved seizure control, 2 remained totally seizure free (during the study period), and the balance of the others remaining in the study (20) experienced a 32 to 45% reduction in both number and severity of their seizures (depending on the CBD dose). **That's huge, and statistically significant by any rational evaluation.** However, 9 people dropped out, due to 'either lack of efficacy or side effects,' which was never clarified; which was actually a potential 18% failure rate. The exact reasons would seem important (if only to avoid speculation), but don't seem to be available about WHY they dropped. However, backed by history, over centuries, the pro- marijuana and pro-CBD oil promoters claim that it's physically impossible to over dose on marijuana or CBD Oil in their natural, normal, forms.

And frankly, we've yet to uncover even one example that they are wrong, using an untainted version of either. The reports are that people 'feel sleepy' or lethargic' but not life threatening. With that said, **caution is still given, because ANY ADDITIVES could be a potential problem**, and few things are 100% purely and solely 'that' thing... there are carriers, flow agents, cutting agents, dilutions, added or extra ingredients, etc. any of which could potentially become a problem, or cause some side effect, depending on the individual and the care given in the manufacturing process.

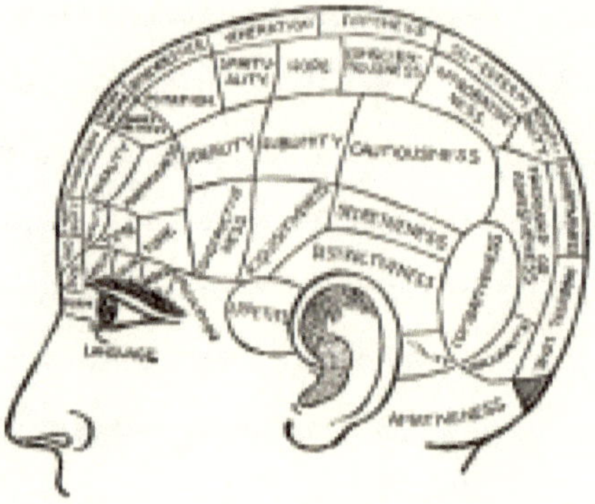

Further, the study didn't offer any real specifics about the 'types' of seizures, frequency, age (other than usually child, usually under 12, at least in the videos released to the public... which may be quite different from the actual study patients). Nor did they discuss the other factors, which could be important to the doctors (and patients) considering their own applications.

While it is a clearly significant breakthrough for that specific group of people, and type of epilepsy, and highly promising for many other brain, nerve, physiological issues... **there really needs to be more numbers and detail in the studies for more doctors to universally accept the information, and be willing to try it on their own patients.**

It's also key to note, that the dose they used was, in Epidiolex, is 100mg/ml... which means there is 10,000mg CBD in the 100ml bottle (3,000mg in 30ml); with only they know which other cannabinoids... and what level and type of THC. This level of potency, in CBD Oil, seems to be a rare find in the consumer market, and would be considered very expensive. (most product we have seen in the consumer market are highly cut, at 100, 300, 500, 1000mg PER BOTTLE… requiring people to DO THE MATH on what it actually is per ml).

PTSD – There are many studies that show a documented 'calming' effect of CBD Oils, but more so when there is also some THC involved, for those that suffer from PTSD and many of the common symptoms associated with that. The study results for this specific issue are why some of the VA Hospitals have decided to overlook some Veterans having THC in their system; though they won't pay for it, or specifically won't prescribe it at this time. (Much more on that later, in the section under 'Insurance and Benefits Concerns')

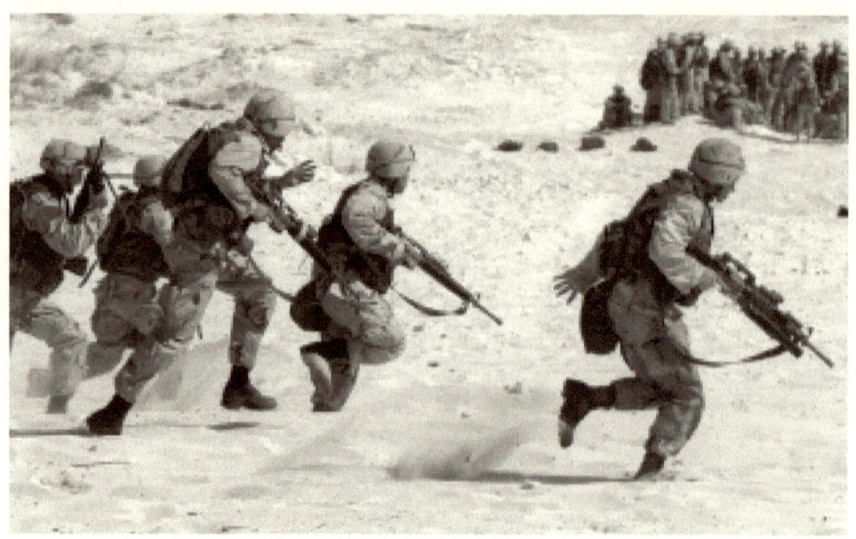

CANCER - There are also some researchers that have shown that CAN help treat, prevent, and even cure **certain types** of brain, breast, and prostate cancers.

There is repeated evidence, by multiple researchers, in unrelated studied, that have found CBD (as well as THC) has a positive impact on some of the symptoms from conventional cancer treatments (like chemotherapy). One of the many findings science has repeatedly learned is that **both THC and CBD** help control (and eliminate) nausea and vomiting, especially among those patients undergoing cancer treatments which usually cause such problems.

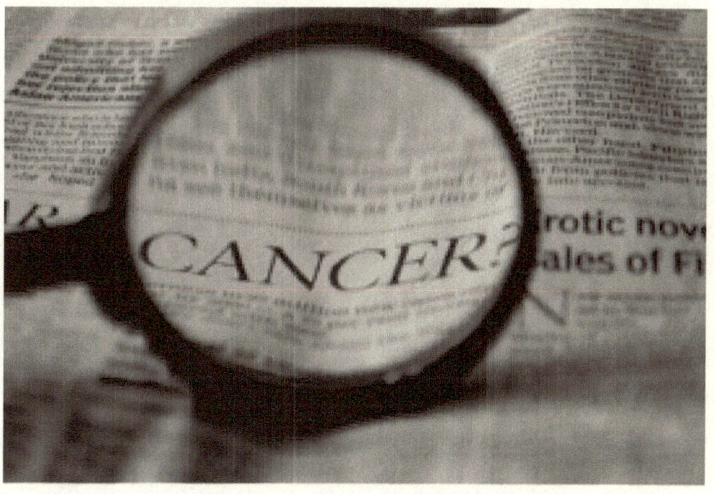

Important note, we couldn't find even one study showing positive effect and success of CURING or TREATING actual cancer without THC also in the mix. Not one. Most successes used a 50:50 ratio, equal portions of THC: CBD, and then often using a specific type of Cannabinoid, targeting a specific type of cells, or having a specific purpose. So those companies claiming all CBD Oil is the same, or JUST CBD Oil 'can do it' (against cancer) probably shouldn't be trusted; unless they really step up and SHOW THE PROOF that THEIR PRODUCT supports their claims. There is more information on this later.

Dr. David Meiri, the lead researcher on the Israeli cancer project, has been studying 50 varieties of cannabis, and their effects on 200 different types of cancer cells. He explains, "There is a large body of scientific data which indicates that cannabinoids specifically inhibit cancer cell growth and promote cancer cell death." He also seems to be a huge proponent of the belief that THC MUST BE combined with CBD Oil to have much hope at fighting cancer cells. Acknowledging that the **treatment is a FULL-SPECTRUM of products**, for the 'entourage effect.'

Co-Factors matter; co-factors are other nutrients & ingredients necessary to make stuff work as completely, correctly, and as bio-available as possible.

In another study, "The investigations documented that the anti-HCC [Hepatocellular Carcinoma] effects are mediated by way of the CB2 receptor. Similar to findings in glioma cells, the cannabinoids were shown to trigger cell death through stimulation of an endoplasmic reticulum stress pathway that activates autophagy and promotes apoptosis. Other investigations have confirmed that CB1 and CB2 receptors may be potential targets in non-small cell lung carcinoma and breast cancer."

See the Dennis Hill, prostate cancer case (apply or believe at your own risk, as we aren't endorsing any of the information, and don't know anything about this specific case, other than what we've read). The presentation appears both interesting and compelling... and worthy of consideration. Mr. Hill used 1gram, split into half doses, twice a day with a 1:1 ratio of THC : CBD for his daily dose.

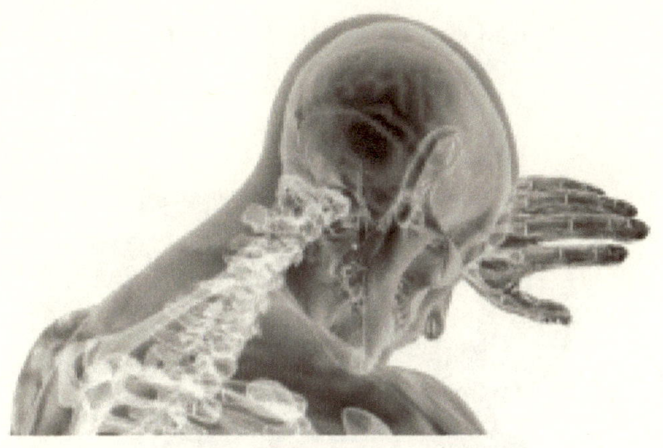

Kelly Hauf, says she used CBD Oil AND THC, to remove a brain tumor. Again, take it with a grain of salt, and with the necessary skepticism, as we don't know the case, the patient, or any of the doctors... only the compelling story being told; and again note: it's BOTH THC and CBD, not one or the other.

Tommy Chong, from movie fame and comedy duo Cheech & Chong, swears that Hash Oil, high in THC and CBD, and a proper diet, cured his prostate cancer. Considering he didn't do chemo or surgery, and his PSA's (Prostate-Specific Antigen) are reported normal with no further sign of cancer… it appears he was 100% correct.

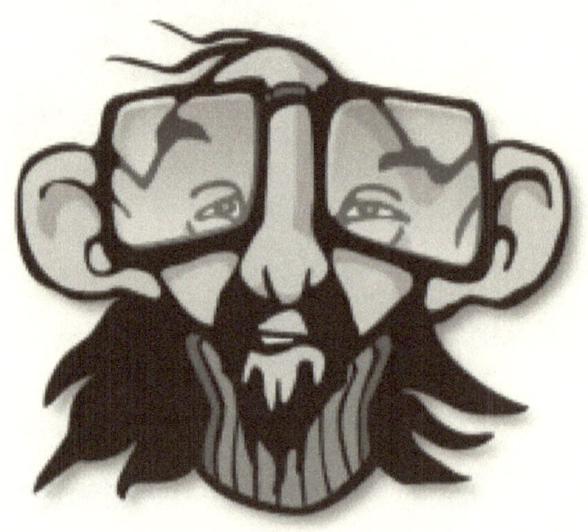

Another Study, conducted in Spain, the researchers used THC and CBD oil to treat cancers successfully. "The International Medical Verities Association is putting **canabis oil on its cancer protocol**. It is on a prioritized protocol list whose top five items are magnesium chloride, iodine, selenium, Alpha Lipoic Acid and sodium bicarbonate. It makes perfect sense to drop cannabis oil right into the middle of this nutritional crossfire of anti-cancer medicines, which are all available without prescription." (Again, note: CANNABIS OIL, with THC & CBD, not 'hemp' oil).

Dr. Abrams, a leading oncologist at University California's UCSF Osher Center, says he has seen cannabis help many with the side effects, but cautions against assuming it is in anyway a cure. He, more specifically said, **"If cannabis definitively cured cancer, I would have expected that I would have a lot more survivors."** No wiser words spoken (or written). However, it's important to understand, according to cancer researchers, only a FEW types of cancer have been 'treated' (helped, reduced, or cured) by some variety of cannabis treatment.

As one doctor reminded us, "research with immunocompetent murine tumor models has demonstrated immunosuppression and **enhanced tumor growth in mice treated with THC."** Another words, for that type of cancer, the use of THC INCREASED the growth of the cancer cells. Working with an educated and experienced doctor is even more important, more vital, could really be the difference between life and death.

There are studies, like the 2015 journal article, in Oncology Reports, showing success in CBD+THC (1:1 ratio) in treating early stages of Prostate Cancer. Another study conclusion showed SLOWING, NOT STOPPING... TREATMENT, NOT CURE "In an in vivo model using severe combined immune deficient mice, subcutaneous tumors were generated by inoculating the animals with cells from human non-small cell lung carcinoma cell lines. Tumor growth was inhibited by 60% in THC-treated mice compared with vehicle-treated control mice."

With more states legalizing it, and the federal government not pursuing convictions as it had been in the past, **we'll be seeing even more actual**

peer reviewed studies, abstracts, and articles getting published in real medical journals… proving and even disproving, speculations and hypothesis that have been discussed in the shadows for years.

SCHIZOPHRENIA – There are piles of anecdotal reports, but also many actual studies on the topic. As one study stated, "A high dose of delta9-tetrahydrocannabinol (THC), the main Cannabis sativa (cannabis) component, **induces anxiety and psychotic-like symptoms in healthy volunteers.**

However, these effects of delta9-tetrahydrocannabinol are significantly reduced by cannabidiol (CBD), a cannabis constituent which is devoid of the typical effects of the plant. **This observation led researchers to suspect that CBD could have anxiolytic and/or antipsychotic actions.**"

Low doses of THC, and higher doses of CBD, seem to have a positive impact on the mental health, and sometimes reducing the amount of pharmaceutical drugs necessary to stabilize moods. This *might* be something to discuss with your mental health provider; as self-medicating can be quite dangerous.

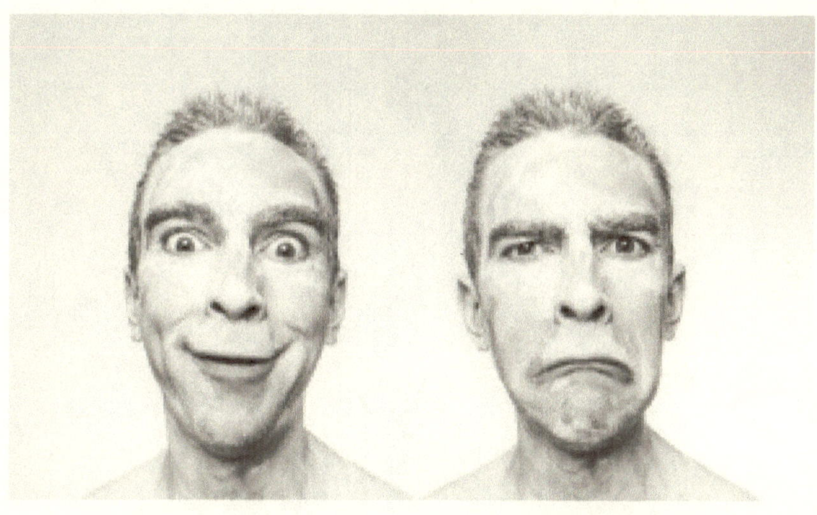

ARTHRITIS – Some studies show pain reduction (aka masking), and some instances of blocking the immune response (which really could be a double edge sword). There is absolutely no proof it helps prevent, heal, cure, or even treat the underlying cause(s) (despite the marketing claims). Science does show that it can have a positive potential in **pain management** and immune system response blocking that might have an impact on RA (rheumatoid arthritis), nothing in cannabis positively helps the body heal any of the actual joint tissue. It will not eliminate or reverse osteoarthritis, though it might help relieve some pain and inflammation. By itself, it allows the cause, **the underlying problem, to get worse.**

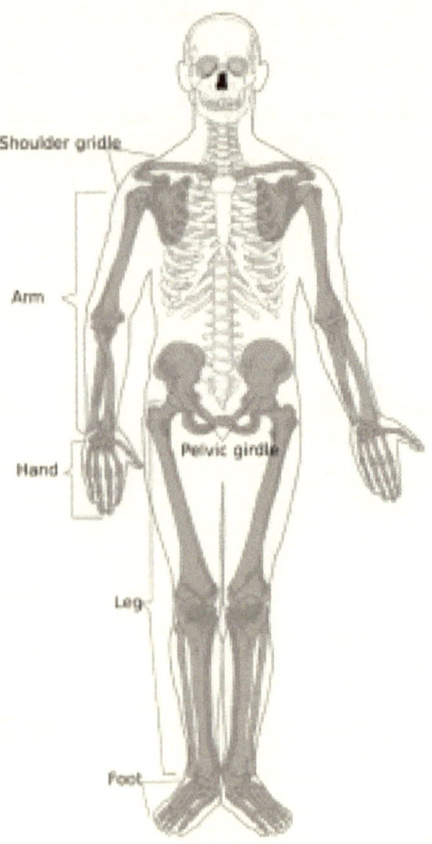

CHRONIC PAIN - There are claims that CBD Oil can reduce chronic pain. This can be significant for those that either can't afford necessary surgery, or such treatment didn't help and find themselves still having chronic pain. Especially for those people over 45 years old, and on a fixed or limited income.

The concept is supported by some science; however, people forget that pain usually occurs for a reason, as a sign of something structurally wrong. Merely **masking that pain doesn't eliminate the underlying problem**, but rather only masks some of the pain... covering up symptoms, allowing the reason there is a problem to actually get worse. This latter fact is grossly ignored in most of the science, which usually limits their research to immediate gratification – reducing pain and improving range of motion (which is usually limited by the pain). The MASKING is often the justification for the misinformation, do by most marketing promoting CBD.

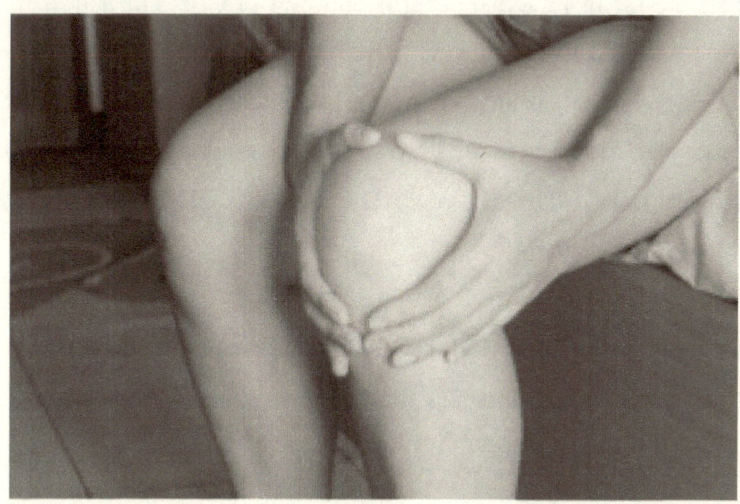

MOOD – It has been shown, repeatedly, to have a direct and reasonably consistent impact on moods. Anti-depressant effects, calming, and even promoting proactive self-preservation and safety type concerns where panic would otherwise normally set in (without the CBD influence).

MAGIC CURE ALL - CBD Oil is NOT a magic cure-all as so many claim; but it does seem to have some real science supporting some of the claims, surrounding certain forms of epilepsy, and Parkinson's, Cancers, and even some chronic pains.

Other areas studies are actively being reported on:

Antitumor Effects –

Antiemetic Effects –

Analgesia -

Sleep Disorders –

There are far more actual benefits and uses of CBD Oil than there ever were for the 'Pet Rock' (another fad, which was never outlawed); however, all the marketing isn't true, honest, or scientifically supported. CBD can impact pain receptors in the nervous system, masking symptoms, there is currently NO EVIDENCE of CBD Oil without THC positively treating any type of cancer.

Pay attention, as some vital information may help you or your loved one in the future. If a companies marketing is pushing medical or healing CLAIMS

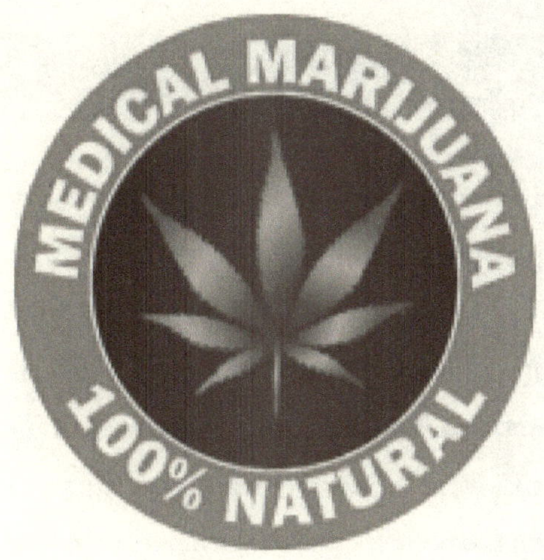

Remember, Poison Oak, Poison Ivy, and Hemlock are 'all natural' plants, that will KILL YOU! Just because it's natural to the world doesn't mean it's good, safe, or helpful to the body. **Mercury is organic, as is asbestos, but they are BAD FOR YOU! Uranium is 100% natural, and medically beneficial (in certain circumstances, and extremely limited and controlled quantities), but too much, or the wrong type will kill you!**

So don't buy into the 'all natural' and 'it's organic' marketing hype! With that said, Cannabis, by itself, in any form, has not yet documented any human death by overdose… however, the synthetic stuff, and some of the herbs added to some of the stuff out there have harmed people… and even killed them! Buyer Beware!

COLORS OF CBD OIL IS TELLING:

The colors and consistency matters, and can tell you a great deal about the quality of the product you're getting.

RAW - is uncut, with only the toxin or impurities in the soil and used in the extraction process. It is dark green in color. If it is 'strong' (high mg per ml) it should NOT be very clear, golden or yellow, in appearance. Industrial Hemp tends to be more brown, and runny (similar to flax seed oil).

DECARBOXYLATED - . It's usually a golden brown to dark brown in color, potentially even almost black in appearance. It has been heated up, cooked or baked. Some say this can increase the potency of THC, when it's included in the oil, because THCA begins to decarboxylated at about 220 degrees Fahrenheit after 30-45 minutes, becoming THC. However, the terpenoids and cannabinoids integrity are compromised at temperatures over 300 degrees Fahrenheit. (Note: CBN is formed by degradation and oxidization of THC). However, an end product could be merely cut with hemp or flax seed oil, to get that brown color.

FILTERED - goes through processing, usually containing any of the same toxins from the soil or processing (as above), but as many of the phytochemicals (THC & THCA) and plant materials are filtered out. Some marketers claim this is the highest quality CBD, and commonly referred to as 'Gold'. It's generally thick, but not quite as thick as honey. We couldn't find a COA on any, for what's actually in it.

CUT – (aka diluted, watered down (just not with water)). Most are 'Cut' and also the easiest to 'fake.' More common when the prices we've seen for the real stuff is in the $150 to 300 range for just 100mg per day dose; which is on the low end of what most of the science calls for to treat serious issues. It happens by unscrupulous, to sell the diluted stuff to the unknowing public. Cutting with almond, coconut, grape seed, fish, or other oils, making it appear more like a 'runny gold.'

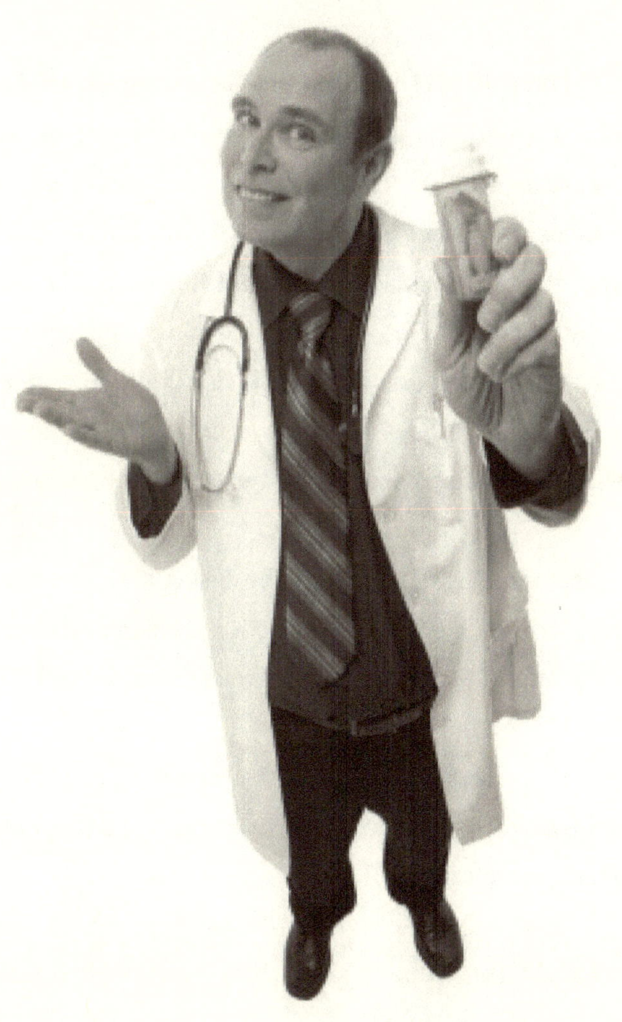

FOUR SENSES – FACTORS TO CONSIDER –

Just exactly what does it FEEL, SMELL, and TASTE like? Those things matter, and can impact the quality, potency, and consistency of the product.

LOOK – Refer to the section on COLORS for more information on this.

SMELL – It should NOT have a strong fishy smell, especially when first opened… especially if it's supposed to be pure. However, all CBD oils priced below about $250 for a 30ml bottle are diluted, with something. The questions are **WHAT** is it cut with, how much, and **what is really in the bottle**? Pay close attention to SHELF LIFE (especially once opened). Some substances have a negative reaction to oxygen, particularly those products with a fish oil base. They start to drastically degrade within about 10 day (generally 30 days maximum after opening), especially if not refrigerated. Be aware, and watch for significant changes to smell or taste.

FEEL – the 'touch' part. In general, the thicker the more pure, usually. It might be a little sticky like real honey, but shouldn't be watery or runny like vegetable oils. It is an OIL, so it should feel a bit 'slick.'

TASTE – it shouldn't taste overly fishy, if it does, that means it's been cut with Fish Oils, and **has to be refrigerated**… and then only has about a 30 day life expectancy.

We've found that some of the best, and most reputable CBD manufacturers generally do testing, for both actual CBD and THC levels in the FINISHED PRODUCT, as well as all the common toxins, pesticides, heavy metals, and microbiological contaminants. Those lab results are shipped with each 'batch' (they have tested), in the form of a COA (Certificate of Analysis). Ask for it when possible, listen to what they say IF they don't supply it. We've found that those who make the results available to buyers, and prospective accounts that have a reasonable reason for their request, are usually the most aware… and most reputable.

POTENCY VARIANCES

Aside from the obvious, milligrams (mg) per dose of x-measurement, knowing the plant source is important. Like different breeds of dogs, cannabis has vastly different features and components, depending on whether the raw material is sativa, indica, ruderalis, or some genetically modified variety or mixture.

Next most important is the labeling on CBD Oil. This is wildly inconsistent, and often deceptive. There are significant differences among formulas, because of the following…

We've seen bottles being marketing from 50mg to 5000mg to consumers. It seems that 100mg, 250, 500, 1000, 2000, and 3000mg are the most common concentrations sold retail. The bottles also have different sizes, 10, 30, 60, 100, and 120ml **seem to be the most common options; usually sold in either 10 or 30ml bottles. Some all-important math is necessary, to determine the amount you are REALLY GETTING.** If there is 3,000mg in a bottle, that works out to 100mg per ml if the bottle is 30ml, but only 12mg/ml if those 3,000mg are in a 250ml bottle. Just 3.33mg per ml if there is only 100mg in a 30ml bottle. Those are huge differences!

The 30ml bottle seems to currently retail for about $35 to $300 a bottle, with actual concentration, potency, cutting agent, testing, and actual components being the primary differences. Eye droppers generally measures 1ml, with a normal squeeze.

However, I've seen bottles labeled xxx mg's… that were never clear where those milligrams claims (and calculations) were coming from, and could only assume it was 'per bottle.' The least concentration, and most common listing method. Especially true with the stuff we've seen being sold in flea markets, swap meets, and some of the on-line companies targeting customers with limited budgets.

Always double check, is the mg listing - per bottle, per oz, per ml, per dropper, per drop, or something else? If you're going to be using this type of product, YOU NEED TO KNOW the math! And be aware; especially if you're hoping to treat anything. It's just as important as knowing ALL OF THE INGREDIENTS.

When cannabis is cultivated for its psychoactive properties, or high THC, male plants will usually be separated from female plants to prevent fertilization. This can facilitate Sinsemilla flowering, or provide control over which male is chosen (to fertilize the female plants). Pollen produced by the male is caught, labeled and stored, until it is needed. Those serious about their cultivation are meticulous about their fertilization process, and plant genetics. Often far more than any other horticulturalists, except maybe some of the specialty show rose or iris growers.

There are some companies pushing the PASTE (over the oil)... claiming it is 'whole plant' derived (seeds, stems, leaves, flowers, and buds), which should actually contain more of the 300 to 500+ different type of cannabinoids and terpenes; but the majority of the paste products we've seen don't have any QA (quality analysis) or CofA (Certificate of Analysis), which is vital to the reality of what is actually in their product.

Entourage Effect Data (also known as 'Synergistic effects' or 'co-Factors') where other 'ingredients, nutrients, or parts are necessary to optimism the effect and ability of the 'Formula' (or the 'medicinal value). The reality is that there are hundreds of other chemical components naturally in the cannabis plant, and they are different, depending on the part of the plant harvested, the soil, and the different strains creates different individual plant character... different acts and actions, not just different 'tastes' or 'smells.'

The chemicals found in cannabis are not just THC or CBD, but actually over 300 to 500 different   cannabinoids, along with other compounds called terpenes and flavonoids. (we'll cover all that in more depth later). The combination of all the components determines what the plant actually does to a body (and the cells within); further focuses on how it does it, and where in the body it impacts the most. It's nearly as diverse as petroleum. **Different cannabinoids react with different cells and receptors in the body;** science has shown them to be quite specific in where they can go (and what they can – and can't – actually do).

A 2018 report in Nature magazine found that actual content of found in cannabis tests varies greatly across consumer products with the same name, and even the same exact product across different testing facilities. This reality is a large part of the problem, and challenge, for commercial growers.

Stay away from non-cannabis herbs used in daily supplement intended for prolonged use (much more information at HerbsAreDrugs.com if interested). The differences exist in consistency, potency, quality, purity, value, effectiveness, and even safety are huge. (especially for Parkinson suffers and Cancer patients) Remember, ZERO actual 'over doses' from real cannabis, over 1,000 from products claiming to be 'like' or herbal.

MANUFACTURING PROCESSES

The problems are quality, consistency, potency, and testing. There currently are no regulations or standardizations in the industry. As you will see, if you look at all the differences that clearly exist, the vast differences in products, claims, and the variety of salespeople trying to cash in.

- Hemp SEED doesn't have any CBD...
- Hemp STEMS, LEAVES, FLOWERS & BUDS do (have CBD)
- Hemp Flowers & Buds have more THC than flower & buds... which is why they are usually avoided, or the cbd is collected from them differently.
- Avoid SEED extracts... (for CBD)

Most CBD, unless it says CANNABIS CBD, or THC+CBD, is derived from hemp if it's being sold on line today, or retail in states marijuana isn't legal for recreational use, because of the absolute limits of the THC (the feds have been cracking down on any that have above 0.3% THC... still, and really).

Today, you'll only touch the real 'cannabis oil' – containing some ratio of THC+CBD in a few of the LEGAL STATES that have active growers & producers (Colorado, Oregon, Washington, maybe California... in particular... everything out of Kentucky, Georgia, and North Carolina right now is INDUSTRIAL HEMP - some there have Federal Research Grow Permits).

The penalty for being wrong falls upon the end-user, no one else. There is no 'lemon law' on CBD product that doesn't accomplish what they claim. The very real fraud laws could be in effect, if people can prove a product actually harmed them (and it wasn't something else they did, which would probably be the defense for those behind a less than perfect, or grossly over sold, product). It's not the grower, manufacturer, persons labeling or even selling the product… without a serious, long, and expensive legal battle. **You, the actual product user, is ultimately responsible for what you choose to put into your body.** And it will be you that has to deal with whatever issue might come up – good or bad, right or wrong, from the use.

The manufacturing process will absolutely influence bioavailability. There are two primary ways CBD OIL is extracted (processed), they are:

1. **Solvent based extraction** This is generally the most common method, and least expensive methods of extracting the oils, is by using solvent. Some are synthetic chemicals, surfactants, and emulsifiers. Some involve nasty toxins, like butane, hexane, pentane, propane, and of course hydrocarbon gases. Because of the nature of the plant, and the process, it is not uncommon (i.e., common) that some of the residuals from these chemicals can end up in the oil and finished product being consumed. These toxins have been traced to issues that compromise the immune system function, and even impede healing.

Some use grain alcohol, or a pharmaceutical-grade ethanol, which are said to kill any bacteria, and even eliminate certain toxins said to commonly exist in some raw plants. However, there are creditable claims this method destroys the plants 'natural' waxes and resins, which drastically reduces potency of key ingredients. It involves allowing solvents to break down the components, and then burning off the solvent, so the oil remains. There are a variety of solvents that can be used, ethanol and butane are used the most often.

If the 'product' is 'white' (odds are), the following things:

1) It is NOT OIL, but a concentrate, of ISOLATED CBD ('cannabidiol')

2) It is JUST CBD (likely 95 to 99.x%) - with no other cannabinoids, which could be significant... depending on what you're using it for.

3) It is under 0.3% THC (likely 0.001% - not generally detectable in standard testing, or in the blood stream) ... because it is 'isolated'

4) Proper dosing is a bit tougher (to calculate) ... because the ENTIRE CONTAINER is xx00mg of straight CBD, so proper measuring may be tough

5) the 'gram' referred to on the product label is likely measured in WEIGHT, not DENSITY, or actual POTENCY, which makes math more challenging (because of the potential purity).

6) because it's 'white' - that means it's likely ETHANOL (solvent) derived processing (not pressed, and clearly not oil).

7) When a product lists CBD with periods between the letters (C.B.D.) a yellow light goes off (in my mind), because the initials do not stand for different words. The only reason I can think a manufacturer would do that is hoping to standout and appear different (alphabetically)..

8) Look for an expiration date... lot number... a manufacturers date... and shelf life estimate, if those are missing, that's a concern (another warning light).

9) when I search for the name on the package - the company or product, and I find NOTHING... I can only assume the company is 'fly by night' (snake oil)... and limiting their liability, by staying off the proverbial grid. Honest, ethical, and LEGAL companies

have website, facebook or google, and other things ON LINE these days. Especially when they are selling through retail stores that could have government officials walk in.

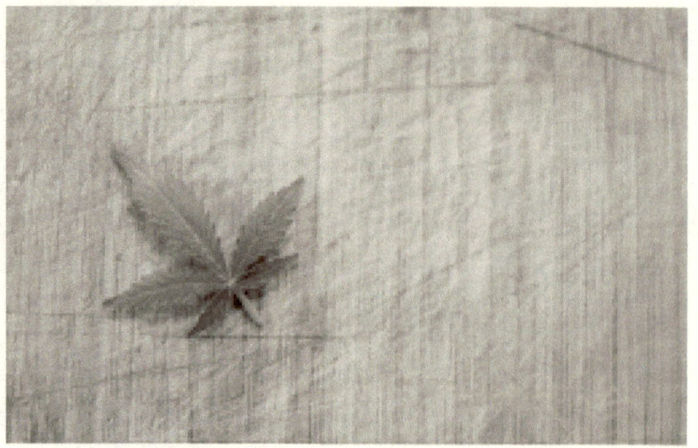

2. **Pressure extraction** has been used for centuries, for flax seed oil, linseed oil, sesame seed oil, peanut oil, etc. etc. Sometimes high temperatures are used, sometimes temperatures are created in the cold processing if things are rushed (from the friction).

   Cold pressing requires the seeds to be 'deshelled' before processing. The outer husk, surrounding the actual seed must be removed before oils are extracted via a cold press.

There is a 'hot press' method, which is also common because it is faster than 'cold pressing,' where CO2 is used (Supercritical or subcritical). It is also a popular alternative to solvent processing. They use high pressure carbon dioxide and low temperatures to isolate the oils. Most of the best seed oil producers agree that it is NOT BETTER than cold processing;, but agree it is way better than solvent processing. It's also been said that food grade oils: olive, coconut, sweet almond, and fish oils can effectively be used in the extraction process. They help keep the friction down, enhance extraction, and infuse the dilution with the extract to a point the oils coming out the other side are pre-mixed. **Certain infused oils, and diluted products,** are absolutely perishable, and should be stores in a COLD, DARK place!

Personally, we believe the cold- pressed method for extraction is generally the best method to extract any oils from any plants or seeds, preserving the maximum amount of nutrients. With cannabis, it doesn't damage the terpenes, flavonoids, or essential cannabinoids from plant. There is a lot of science, over the centuries, from other plant oils manufacturers, which absolutely support cold pressure processing over heat & high pressure, both of which are better than using any solvents. **Pressure processing produces a cleaner, more natural taste, and most all common mycotoxins cannot survive the processing.**

Sadly, it seems to be more like the 'gold rush' for many manufacturers, with many passing off iron pirate (fool's gold), or low quality gold riddled with impurities. While there seems to be serious science and a whole lot of potential for quality CBD oil, the reality is they aren't all the same, though they share the same name. It is just another 'snake oil' scheme in many cases; for some, it's the latest MLM (multi-level marketing) pyramid scheme for those hoping to 'get rich quick' off those suffering.

Any of the following things can drastically change a 'batch' of finished product, creating very real differences in concentration, potency, function, effectiveness, and toxins. Even between shipments, and between the same exact 'formulas' from different companies.

- Source for raw materials (species of raw materials)
- Harvest (same species in different soils, times of year)
- Production methods (solvent vs pressure – hot vs cold)
- Processing Method and procedures
- Diluents used
- Bottling and packaging controls & methods
- Shipping/delivery methods
- Storage & dispensary procedures
- How it's used…

Each of those factors will impact quality, potency, and even the shelf life of the product. Ultimately the usefulness of a product to the person seeking benefit. Just like honey can have a different flavor, depending on what the bees eat... the same exact species of cannabis can be varied based the soil, climate (indoors or outdoors), and even the pollination methods. They are each and all reflected in the final product.

CBD Oil has tested out from 0.001% THC, which is great if you're looking to avoid THC), but ugly expensive. There is more than is <0.3% THC, which is still very good, but often also lacks the actual CBD's... and can be considered expensive, but not as expensive as the first example. Neither of these are likely to be traceable in blood tests, with normal use levels. HOWEVER, some products labeled as low or no CBD Oils have also tested out with as much as 3 to 5% THC, despite their label claims (which could easily be a problem).

It's also important to know that some of the manufacturing processes can be dangerous, not just to those making the product... but even more so to the unsuspecting end-users buying unethical, untested, and tainted product.

There are far safer methods, that don't use any chemicals... the most common is COLD PRESSING.

Be aware of 'window dressing' (on labels, in marketing & advertising, and sales) of CBD products)... things like 'gluten free' – omega fatty acids – superfood – zero THC – 100% pure – 100% THC FREE – high in vitamin E, etc. etc. etc. Watch for truth and lies, and actual science.

The reality is that the gray zone created between the legal states, limited enforcement by the federal government, and the 'gold rush' mentality of those wanting to make some quick cash… has invited a whole lot of shady characters, actual crooks, as well as some good people just looking to make some money more easily. The general lack of knowledge, promise of the 'magic pill' (as it were), and missing regulations (by the government or industry) has moved the black market to main stream. Amazon and eBay, most flea markets, swap meets, and farmers markets have one to ten plus people pushing products claimed to be CBD oil. Some really have some amount (tested), but many are diluted or just plain fake. Even more are mislabeled. It doesn't require much critical thinking to realize it's been a market filled with both good people that mean well, as well as major crooks and con-artists.

Quality, whole plant efficacy, can absolutely and medically help some things, and have scientifically proven to have outstanding and amazing health benefits for some things, **but not everything!** Read on, to learn common reasons why….

Page Intentionally Left Blank for Your Own Notes:

THERE'S GOLD IN CBD & CANNABIS

Well, not in the literal sense, but in the 'chance to get rich' sense of the term, it's better than a lotto ticket. How it is being marketed, the similarities between the California Gold Rush and the Legalize Cannabis, so people can grow, sell, use, is unmistakably similar. For many, the entire 'legal pot' crusade is even referred to as the modern 'gold rush. It's being sold to 're-sellers' (and investors) as 'an opportunity' that virtually anyone, with a safe place to grow some plants thinking they might make easy money, regardless of their education level, class, race, vocational training, or other factors commonly associated with 'making a living' or 'getting ahead.' If you don't want to grow, no big deal, you are re-sell the finished product to your family and friends, and existing customers, and make money. Much like prohibition and moonshiners.

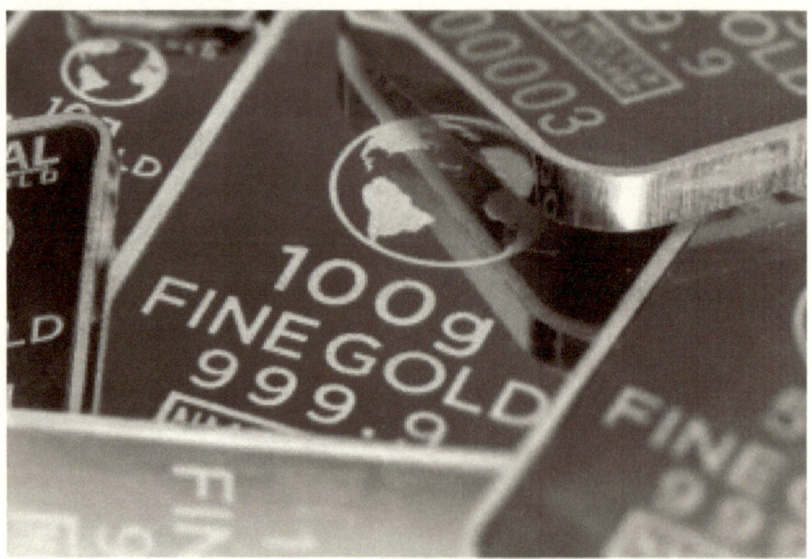

During the prohibition, the price of marijuana could have been more than $5,000 per pound. Today, it is reportedly under $1200 a pound, including the addition of the high taxes most states require sellers to collect. There has been a huge decline in the sales price of marijuana, because of the vast number of growers, and speed in which it grows, and the inability to cross state lines (legally) in most cases and states. The supply is massive, and the demand limited to the citizens in that general area. Sellers staying 'within' state lines, generally 'stay' under state laws. The moment they cross state lines, it can quickly and technically become Federal. That is what most people want to avoid.

However, the cost of concentrated CBD oils are high, and unlikely to go down anytime soon… despite the often undisclosed, misleading purity levels, quality, potency, and benefits claims. It is actively being shipped across state lines… even sold on Amazon, eBay, and a wide variety of internet websites.

CBD Oil is usually being sold as a 'cure all' and 'mother nature's answer' for just about anything and everything that ails you. The problem is that only a few things have been proven, some have been disproved, and many are still untested, unverified, or poorly studied.

CBD Oil is much the same as gold. They are both sold with an illusion of need, through an emotionally charged offer of solutions. Gold is the 'bling' the illusion or example of class, success, worth, or value. CBD is the illusion of health, healing, or cures. Both are designed to sell, at a variety of price points, with the marketer's belief that 'something' is better than nothing. The problem is the number of products out there that, like gold, are marketed as 'pure' – 100% - zero THC – that are really just 'gold plated' or a fraction of the real deal.

Same as there is no such thing as 100% 'pure gold.' At best, it is 99.9% at most, and that's only for 24k (karat). Step down to 22k gold, and there is only 91.67% actual gold. 18k is just 75% real gold (25% copper, silver, zinc, or potentially other metals). **14k is just 58.3% actual gold**, 12k is only 50%, **10k is only 41.7%** actual gold, and that 'gold plated' stuff… well, it is LESS THAN 1% actual gold!

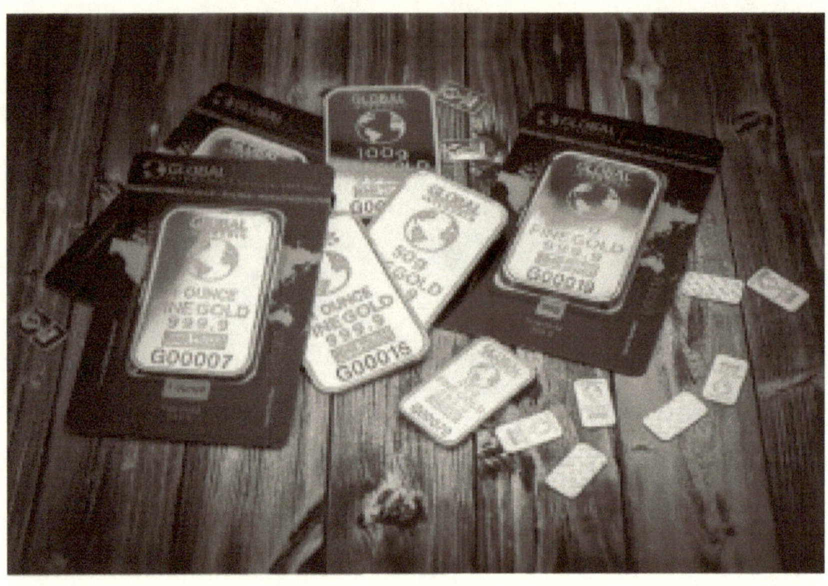

Remember, the 'placebo effect' works on about 20% of the population, so even the garbage stuff will have believers and followers. You can believe the majority of the researchers aren't using the fake stuff, or low quality cheap stuff for their studies, experiments, or tests. They are focused on mg/ml… usually with 2 or 3 applications a day, and usually with some pretty strict parameters. It is important to understand WHAT THEY DID/USED to get the results… and precisely what those results were.

Less pure stuff usually has a much greater profit. Herbs are often added to give a false, but usually real fast sense of 'it is workings.' (By masking some symptoms).

There are significantly different quality levels. Except, with gold, it is generally MARKED, with a standardized set of numbers, that mean essentially the same thing, regardless where you purchased that gold. Buying 14k gold from 10 different places, you can rest assured that you'll be getting 58.3% actual gold minimum for all 10 places. It is basically a color or hardness difference, a conductivity difference, which impacts the cost and value difference with some 'standards' anyone buying or selling gold can easily learn, and understand. Today, the same can't be said about CBD products, even many of them with claimed mg's.

There is a whole lot of 'marketing magic' and hype, surrounding cannabis products trying to cash in on some quality science that likely doesn't apply to 'that' product, or the level and type of ingredients 'it has.' Mostly it is just because of the 'name' recognition, regardless what it is really made of, what is actually in it…

Caveat Emptor – Buyer Beware. Learn to ask the right questions, and how to determine who you can actually trust, who can't, and why.

As a joker on Facebook pointed out on an advertisement on fakebook, "My sister had her arm amputated in a car accident. Three years later, she started using CBD. After 6 months her arm grew back. I'm saying this on FB, so that means it's true." - Marc Maksim. The post he put that comment on was making grandiose and false claims, which any educated person that had done the slightest research could spot.

Yes, there really is science, and a whole lot of medical researchers and real doctors, with published peer reviewed studies, which show statistical significances and benefits for treating some types of epilepsy, some types of cancer, some types of chronic pain (especially spinal), many different nervous disorders, mental challenges, and some cases of PTSD; but **it is not a 'cure all.'**

It is absolutely a miracle, effective treatment, and medical benefit for SOME THINGS. **Science has demonstrated it is pretty amazing, promising, and enlightening in some areas.** It was some of that very science that caught our attention, and our hope. Which is what makes it so easy to mislead, misdirect, and oversell the product(s), that don't actually meet or match the concentration or potency, or formulas, actually used in the positive science. But people feel hopeful; because they want to believe, and have hope, in effective treatment, and cures... especially when they haven't found it in modern medicine.

Be sure to check out the science for the specific issue you are looking into. Pay attention to, and purposefully look at the numbers, how many bodies were actually involved, how long it lasted, who funded it, and exactly what the specifics were – to the dosing, type, and results.

All science we've found related to cancer involved THC also, not just CBD; and in some cases, it wasn't just THC and CBD that impacted the cancer cells, but one (or more) of the other cannabinoids found in the plant. More importantly, they did not impact all types of cancer, but seem to lessen most all the negative symptoms from conversional cancer treatments. It did have huge promise for some types of cancer (mostly brain, prostrate, and breast). More information later…

For many, especially in the 'legal' states, it is either a 'hopeful fix' if they have a problem (if they are a buyer) or 'free money' (if they are a seller). Either way, it often offers some hope to anyone that otherwise might not think they have much hope or success elsewhere, regardless which side of the proverbial coin they find themselves on. It seems to be of particular interest to those suffering from a chronic illness, or would prefer to 'work from home.' Black market sales are always under the table, and tax free… with the obvious risks. Safer than most prescriptions.

The industry is riddled with ignorance, misinformation, unawareness, inexperience, over generalization, twisted words, lies, wrong interpretations, and legal wrangling. **The unknown, and blind hope, are exactly why unscrupulous and ignorant people started claiming things were legal, when they aren't.**

Some people created fake products hoping to profit from the craze; while the proverbial hemp is hot; knowing their product won't really do what they claim. Many are modern day snake oil salesmen, using the science of other people's product to sell their proprietary concoctions, based on partial truths or complete lies.

Some products seem to be the real deal, but many aren't. Telling them apart can be a real challenge. Tons of awful and completely fake products, thousands of real scams and outright marketing lies pushing false hope and fantasy, all in the name of 'Miracle of CBD's.'

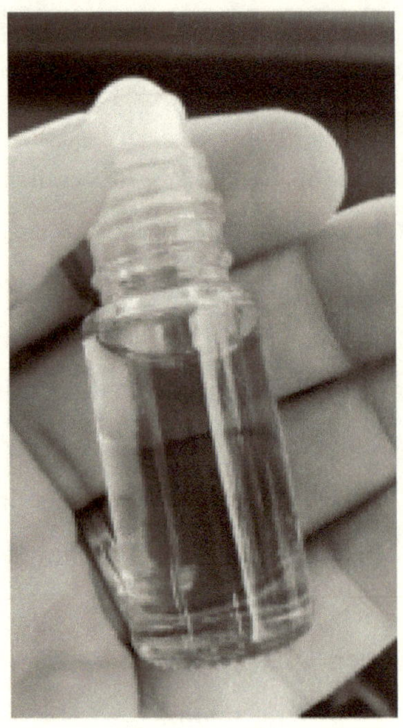

It only goes to reason, that the states that ignored federal laws have produced the most hemp. In 2017, states reportedly licensed more than 39,000 acres for hemp production (countless acres are unregistered, and illegal product is still entering the country). It is unclear how many acres were approved for marijuana production, since not all states require licensing or reporting. Some states only allow academia or select individuals to 'legally' grow with permits or licenses. And the majority are not yet set up to really deal with regulating what they consider it the proverbial beast.

However, some of the differences in cannabis products are because of ignorance, some unscrupulous companies just trying to take advantage of the 'gold rush,' like selling iron pyrite and calling it 'gold.' Not really caring about truth and ethics, just using 'words' the name, and making false claims to promote a product that really isn't 100% 'legal' and doesn't really have 0% THC. **Or they are selling something that wasn't made from any cannabis product to begin with,** might fall under DSHEA with some herbal concoction of pain blockers and neural stimulants, which aren't really safe.

Consider, the CBD Oil Industry sprouted from virtually nowhere, and was less than $10 million just three or four years ago. Initially started, in an attempt to get the benefits cannabis offered, without the THC or smoking (which many were against, attempting to equate cannabis smoke with cigarette smoke). Those promoting it were hoping to get federal approval.

After the video of the epileptic child, Charlotte Figi, being so drastically (and visually) helped. The popularity and sales of CBD oils (particularly a brand named 'Charlotte's Web'), the industry quickly jumped to over $190 million reported in 2017. Her story was told to congress, and was "the girl who is changing medical marijuana laws across America,"

Some estimate that by 2022 it will be pushing over $20 Billion (yep, with a B). Most project cannabis being one of the hottest topics in the 2020 elections (pro vs con, medical vs recreational, legal vs regulated vs banned vs outlawed still).

It's projected that the Cannabis and CBD Industry will sky rocket to over $200 Billion within a year of WHEN it is federally legal, and officially removed as a Schedule 1 controlled substance at the federal level! However, will it remain sustainable?

Many believe it could be a great investment, and the next Google, Microsoft, or other huge stock potential, as long as business managers do their job, and pay attention to laws, stay in compliance, are honest, with good product ... it really could be an amazing investment, so long as it's 'pure' stuff, without any other herbs or synthetics, or wrong additives.

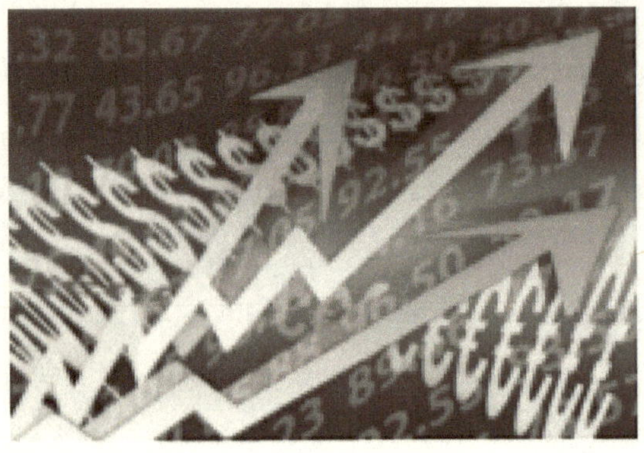

With all the medical break-throughs, and science showing positive effects and treatment of a variety of issues, it appears that the question isn't 'IF' it becomes 100% legal federally, but WHEN it is officially decriminalized (at least to a similar position as alcohol, with obvious and necessary exceptions).

The Presidential candidate, incumbent or opponent, which promotes legalization and having it removed from the Schedule 1 list, will have millions of easy votes, for no other reason than all those citizens that want the choice, chance, and opportunity to see if it can help them – or their loved one in 2020/24. It will be interesting to see what President Trump does on the topic, if anything; and where all his haters go with that if he comes out to DECRIMINALIZE all cannabis products at the Federal level. Mind you, that's not the same as 'legalize' – it just puts things back into the hands of the individual states. If the citizens of that state don't like the laws, they can move to a state that has the laws they value and want.

Like it or not, cannabis is here to stay, until the end of time, regardless what the government does (or doesn't do), it will continue. Just like Moonshine, jay-walking, and speeding down the highway; and cannabis is statistically safer than all of those. The stats show that over a five-year period, just 1.8 percent of fatal crashes involved drivers who tested positive for cannabis, most of those also tested for alcohol and/or prescription drugs… or were found to suffer from long term mental illness issues.

Be aware of the stats, and who is telling them. Learn to ASK QUESTIONS, and see what is missing when claims are made. WHAT ELSE was involved?

Legality is on the horizon, which is a reality… and just a matter of time, legislation, regulation, safety, and decriminalization.

ZERO % THC

One product label we evaluated: '________ CDB Tincture 3000 mg 0% THC". (Company name omitted, for obvious reasons) Yet, on the back side under the directions, it says "_____ Oil 99%+ pure CDB Isolate."

That means that, really, 99% of that product is a FILLER, a diluent, something other than a cannabis base; with just 1% being the 'CBD Isolate' – which is implied was the entire 3000mg of CBD. That was a 30ml bottle, which means that 1% (all 3000mg) was in just 0.3ml of that bottle, 1/3rd of the standard eye dropper, in 29.97ml of some diluent oil. Wrap your head around that. There is more flavoring on popcorn in the movie theater!

Upon looking further, we learn that extract is claimed to be "extracted from hemp grown under the Kentucky Department of Agriculture Industrial Hemp Research Pilot Program, which was established under the guidelines provided by Section 7606 of the Agriculture Act of 2014(7 U.S.C 5940)" and reports that **"What extract without THC" really means is that when tested, their extract has UNDETECTABLE amounts of THC [with the testing method they used].**

In reality, undetectable still does NOT mean Zero. It means that there is a fraction of a percent, usually .001% to 0.3% THC. Which would be expected when the entire bottle contains just 1/3rd of an eye dropper of 'CBD Isolate,' and THC is just a small fraction of that. Just one example of why basic math is important.

In addition, it means when they chose to test, in the fashion they tested, with the test they selected, did not detect any THC. However, the 'true' amount would depend on HOW it was tested, WHEN it was tested (in RAW or after bottling); and what they tested. Because, if it was tested BEFORE processing, the results would very likely change the after bottling. How 'mixed' were the raw materials, if the testing was done prior to bottling? Some THC stills exists in the finished product, albeit a fraction of a percent (and very probably under 0.3%). Considering their claim that there is 3000mg of CBD in just .3 ml of that product, it's highly likely there is undetectable THC; AND frankly it might even be undetectable CBD's as well. The math is simple, 1% of a 30ml container is 0.3ml... not even an entire single eye dropper of the CBD isolate in the bottle. There was also no proof, or COA, or a list of which of the over 500 cannabinoids were really in their 'CBD isolate.'

The question is what stage was the testing done? Was it raw, or after the extraction, after blending (with the diluent), after bottling, or at some other stage? What ALL was really tested for? If it was done on the 'raw' plants... what part of the plant, how random and accurate is it? Seeds and stems usually have the least amount of THC, so 'undetectable' there... in dried seeds, will not produce the same results as the stems, leaves, buds or flowers,; a 'wet' product (freshly harvested, vs hung upside down for the 'sap' to drain into the leaves, buds, and flowers) will be different than dried plant content.

Note: this labeling has NOTHING TO DO WITH KENTUCKY, or the Research Program. There is no guarantee that the label is honest, or what part(s) of the Industrial Hemp, were even actually used... or if there was any actual testing for CBD's, or any other cannabinoids, in that 1/3rd of an eye dropper that was put in the 30ml bottle.

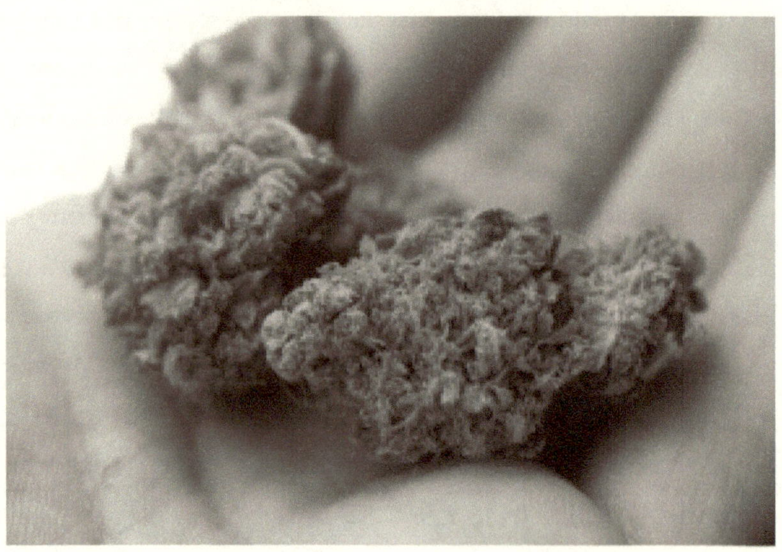

Just like there really is no such thing as 100% pure gold or silver, or that McDonald's puts just 3 pickles on their burgers 100% of the time... **it's all marketing hype, not 100% reality.**

At upwards of $150 a month (for the average, non-epileptic, non-cancer treatment, levels necessary)... and the marketing hype isn't 100% honest, though **some high-end products seem promising**, none of the low end products we've seen appear to be all that honest. Ask for a COA (Certificate of Analysis) and **DO THE MATH!**

If the concerns are seizures, certain cancers, or severe chronic pain, are involved I'd absolutely consider trying it... but the right type, and at the right dosing. Especially IF I was told I have cancer, or a serious issue and wasn't getting any federal benefits. If, however, I was getting such benefits, or had a job that did regular drug testing, OR had a job that could easily or reasonable be considered somehow dangerous, I would absolutely stay away from it, unless I had their approval IN WRITING or was willing to gamble those benefits.

The struggle is trusting anything that claims 100%, yet fails to have proof. Ultimately, it's your life, your illness, your pain, and risking your benefits.

Let's take it all back to the basics. **All cannabis related products utilize an extract from either industrial hemp or marijuana. Both have THC,** though hemp naturally has a level of many of the cannabinoids, even THC, hemp doesn't have ALL of the key cannabinoids. So, to make the claim there is a hemp extract product with "no THC", the THC would have to be removed OR isn't not really a cannabis based product. **If it's derived from the seeds, CBD would have to be added** (because there isn't any CBD in hemp seeds).

You should question the materials used, processing technique, and type of plant(s) it comes from. Reality is the growers have developed a strain of hemp that is naturally ALMOST and MOSTLY 'free of THC,' but still not completely, 100%.

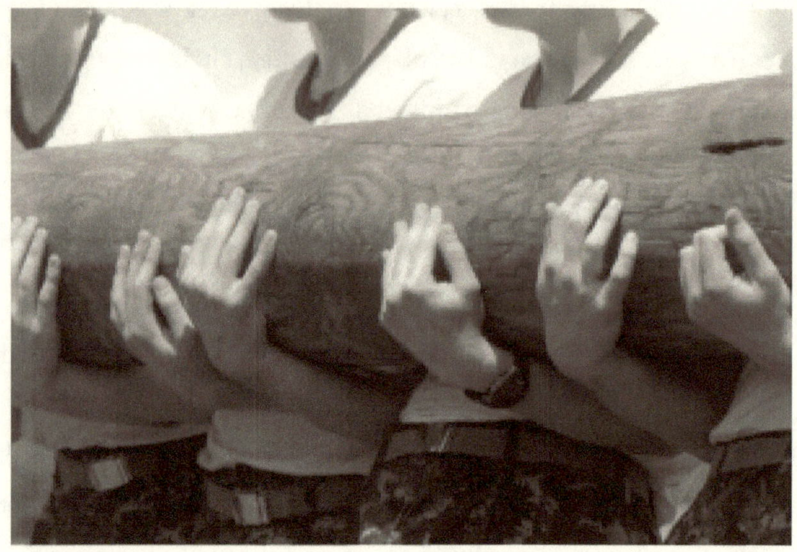

This false claim of '0%' is actually being said quite a bit these last few months. Some are feeling comfortable with that claim, due to the government supposedly over looking for THC levels <0.3%. If the number is below that, the resellers believe the government is 'looking the other way' (sometimes). Except when they don't.

Consumers have been demanding a product they can use, without breaking the law, without any THC (wrongly believing it is JUST CBD that has the medicinal benefits). The majority doesn't want to smoke it, so CBD Oil was created.

The manufacturer's hoped that if the THC levels were low enough, or if it was for medical use… or they are in a 'legal state' – or buying from a grower with a USDA/DEA/FDA 'Industrial Hemp Research Pilot Program' they won't have to worry about any legal problems.

Consumers hoped CBD would be a 'magic fix' for their ailments, cure their problems, and extend their life. However, the reality is that it is like thinking the only liquid a car needs to operate is gas, forgetting about oil, water, antifreeze, brake fluid, transmission fluid, etc. There is more to the science the JUST CBD Oil in most cases.

DOES ANY OF THIS MATTER?

Anyone with common sense, and the slightest research, knows with 30 states already legalizing marijuana, including edibles and CBD Oils by default. It stands to reason that there would be a significant increase in usage… especially as more states legalize it. We know most main stream national media tends to be bias, promoting agendas these days, and they aren't always the best source of news. However, according to a September 7th, 2018, article in CNN Wire, the use of actual marijuana is really exploding, and more people are coming out of the proverbial 'closet.'

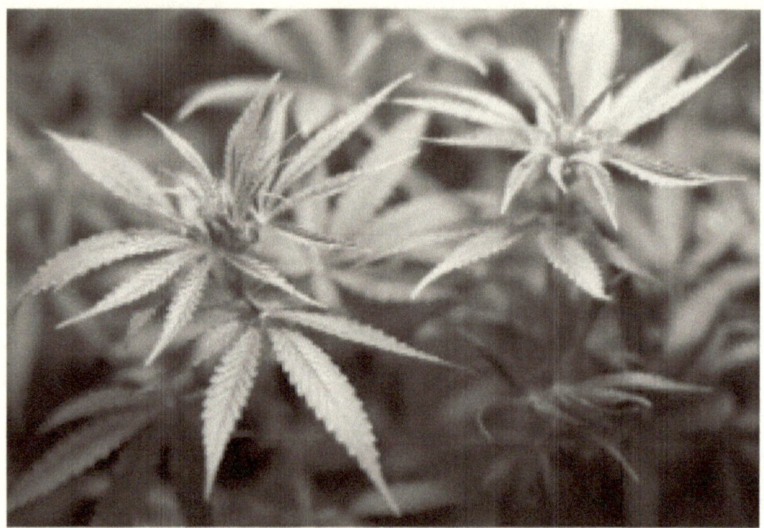

They were more specially referencing a new study reported in the Journal of Drug and Alcohol Dependence, **which examined 17,608 adults 50 and older.** The National Review, tasked with gathering and analyzing data with as little political bias as possible, released their findings. The results demonstrated that older adults (those over 50) have experienced a seven hundred percent (700%) increase in marijuana use over the preceding decade. At that time, they estimated about 9% of the adults between 50 – 64 years old had used marijuana at least once within the previous year, while about 3% older than 65 had used during that same period.

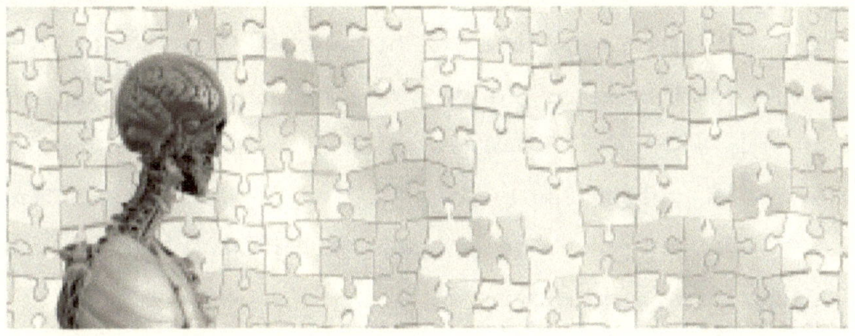

Dr. Benjamin Han was the lead author of the study, and assistant professor at the New York University School of Medicine. The study also showed nearly 5% of that 'middle age' group also had 'alcohol problems; 9% nicotine dependent, and 3.5% misused opioids. For the 'over 65' group, the abuse numbers were 3.5% nicotine, 1.5% alcohol, and 1.2% for misuse of opioids, respectively.

Some other interesting points, were:

- 'baby boomers' (those that were teenagers in the 60's and 70's) were, more than half (nearly 55%) likely to have used marijuana at some point in their lives, while the numbers were just 22% for over 65 group.

- However, **more than half of those that hadn't used before ASKED** their healthcare provider, or a trusted family member or friend, IF THE SHOULD TRY marijuana to help with sleep or chronic pain. Which brings the total up to $(55+(45\%/2))=$ **77.5% willing to consider** and/or use cannabis for medical purposes; particularly for neurological issues, cancer, or chronic pain.

- other reports estimated nearly 80% of the people over 50 are either actively trying CBD Oil or marijuana, or have inquired about trying one or the other, because **they are told it is 'legal.'** They saw some positive science, and remember back to their youth, before most hard or 'bad' drugs hit small towns, and they incorrectly believe it is the 'same' (as that from their youth in the 50's-70's).

- CBD and Hemp Oils are advertised on Amazon, eBay, Facebook; it's on tv more, as well as being pushed in flea markets, at swap meets, discussed in the news, including magazines. **People are being wrongly told that it is all 'ok' and 'totally legal' now** ('in all 50 states' many claim). Therefore, it must be legal and ok now, right? No… it's not, really.

- It is technically illegal on the federal level, and claims stating otherwise are 100% false, as of today! It currently UNENFORCED, generally, which is a far cry from specifically 'legal' or 'legalized,' which is significant; especially if you are arrested or end up with some type of legal challenge.

All edible, smoke-able, topical, and potentially medicinal Cannabis products, including CBD Oil, are still listed as a Schedule 1 Controlled Substance though the federal government, at this time. The DEA's memo May 2018 is purposefully vague, but **does not specifically change anything**. Remember, people still drive 80, 90, 100+ miles per hour in many geographies in this nation…, and get away with it, for a time. Some, for a long time. That does not mean it is legal. In some areas, and times of the day (or night), depending on the traffic flow and other variables, you might even see someone actually speeding passed a police officer that seems to just ignore them… but that still doesn't make it legal. Unenforced laws are not decriminalized… and have not suddenly become legal. When it comes to any actual cannabis products, you are technically committing a crime worse than just speeding… and actually breaking federal laws. That is 100% fact, in America, as of October 9th, 2018!

Now that we have dealt with some of the reality about the truth in legalities, despite what some friend might have told you, or that person at the flea market or in a store… Let's look at **WHAT IT REALLY DOES IN THE HUMAN BODY**, and why. **There really is a lot of awesome science out there, but some junk science too.**

IS IT SAFE?

This is honestly another loaded question.

There has NOT been any actual documented overdoses from pure cannabis, either 'just' marijuana or true CBS Oil that we were able to find… documented anywhere, from any continent, over centuries.

Researchers have pointed out that, because cannabinoid receptors are **not located in the brainstem** areas controlling respiration or the heart beating, lethal overdoses do not occur from Cannabis and cannabinoids. No one has even really smoked or eaten too much actual cannabis product. Nothing saying it caused anyone's death – short term, or even after years of regular use; even at high levels. There are people hoping to push or imply some dangers, some over dose effect, but science does not support those assertions. Any such speculation is not based on any history or reality. It's wishful thinking, on their part, because scientifically it is impossible… with toxin free natural cannabis. At the same point, the potency of cannabis from over twenty years ago vs today is also drastically different, and that shouldn't be ignored.

There are at least two different studies that show the prolonged used of HIGH THC strains of marijuana can change the way developing brains actually grow.

Today, there is also a direct and absolute difference between delivery methods. How much makes it into the body (bio-availability) when used sublingually (under the tongue), vs rectal administration, vs smoked, vs vaped, or eaten (even differences in potency of the same product, when cooked, or baked, vs raw). **Each method of delivery would necessarily have a different (level) of bio-availability and absorption with the same exact 'starting amount.'**

THC is "rapidly absorbed" through lungs after inhalation and "quickly reaches high concentration in blood," once it goes through the lungs, oxygenated by the air you breathe, it gets to the brain quickly. However, when marijuana is consumed in edible forms, it can have longer-lasting effects. Because it is mostly metabolized by the liver, which reduces the overall amount of THC that enters the bloodstream. One study showed that "Ingesting edibles introduces only 10% to 20% of THC, CBD, and other cannabinoids to the blood plasma, whereas INHALED cannabis falls closer to 50% or 60% range" according to Leafly.

Yes, there have been reports of kids getting in to brownies and other edibles, and eating enough they were taken to the hospital, because they 'were lethargic' and 'sleepy' and their care giver was worried, and didn't want anything bad or wrong to happen to the child. Hospital staff merely observed, the children all were fine. Better care of where edibles are kept, and what their children get into, is necessary. Today, it is unknown just how much concentrate (of either THC or CBD) might become dangerous (to anyone). **Children HAVE BEEN KILLED by synthetics!**

Remember, for the nay-sayers, people died from angle dust (PCP), and other substances, sprayed on (or added to) marijuana over the years. Albeit rare, people have also really died from too much water, and far more have died from tainted water. Remember, while too much alcohol can be dangerous (alcohol poisoning), drunk actions, there are far more that have died from chronic long-term alcohol abuse (sclerosis of the liver and other complications) than from any real cannabis product. History doesn't show anyone – not one person - that has ever actually died from cannabis overdose, or even above normal use at home.

However, with that said, understand there are over 1,000 deaths a year, because of unscrupulous companies selling synthetic and other herbs 'AS marijuana' and CBD. Many of these fake products have an actual history of harming people, over 1,000 deaths a year!

Some are claiming there is a potential for COPD (the lung disease) from smoking marijuana, though we found no science supporting that claim... even on daily users. Those making the claim attempt to equate the smoking of pot to cigarettes, and either willfully or ignorantly neglect to acknowledge the fact that 'tobacco' itself wasn't the 'major problem' – but rather the chemicals added to the tobacco. That's not to imply smoking cigarettes is good, but rather than there are huge differences in the TYPE, quantity, frequency, amount inhaled, and even whether it's ventilated.

There are no RDIs (Recommended Daily Intake), or standardized serving size(s), suggested potency levels, or standardized tests for ALL ingredients, listing qualities, known toxins actually in a product, or formula. That NEEDS TO HAPPEN!

Even the government regulated legal marijuana, in the states where it was approved (to grow for testing purposes), **large amounts tested positive**

for herbicidal toxins. Perfectly delicious sounding edibles tested positive for toxins from irresponsible, hurried, or unprofessional people (bad soil or additives). These toxins and heavy metals should be of more concern, and are scientifically more likely to be a problem for the average person than the natural cannabis itself.

If there were responsible tests, and reasonable federal guidelines, and consistency in labeling, that was quick – easy – and affordable, there would be hope. However, without some rational 'self-regulation' and honest reporting within the fast growing industry, it will only take one or two screw ups to make things impossible.

The answer really depends on the safety and process of the growers, harvesters, processors, and manufacturing producers. How careful (and aware) are they?

Without any regulation, aside from how many plants do they have, how much product they are producing, and are they paying all the permit fees and taxes they should… most states don't care about the rest of the stuff, so long as the product isn't quickly killing people. As of today, any and all testing is up to the manufacturer (then only those wanting to justify or prove their quality), the bottler/seller (wanting to limit their liability), or (most often) some third party looking to stop (or block) the legalization (and usually selectively publicizing the results).

If the producers are not careful, their industry could become riddled with over regulations, driving the time to comply, and money costs, up even higher. You might ask the manufacturer if they have a QA (quality analysis) or COA (certificate of analysis) for that particular lot they'd be willing to show, email, or fax you. Some will, most won't – because it should contain some proprietary information about their strain, their formula, what makes their product unique. They are even less likely to share this information if they don't know you, or think you might be a competitor. But more sadly, some won't have a clue what you're talking about, as they don't do any testing. As an end-user, that might be an important piece of information to have.

We've heard of everything from 100mg per bottle, to 100mg per dropper, edible, per capsule, and even per drop. There is no real consistency. Often little or nothing on bio-availability of the CBD Oil concentrates, or cutting agents, or how many actual milligrams of which active ingredients, or other cannabinoids, are proven to actually be in the product listed on most labels. The math is important!

In 2015 through 2019 the FDA took some brands and manufacturer's to task, to set an example (and remind them it's not all open season, even in legal states, and even with the Farm Bill, many things are still not federally legal... just 'Industrial Hemp' and NO THC product not making claims have been federally decriminalized), when they tested products claiming to contain CBD, had none found (neither was there any THC in those products), as the products weren't created from any species of cannabis plants (or their parts), which is fraud!

In general, because cannabinoid receptors are present in tissues throughout the body, not just the brain and central nervous system, there may be some adverse effects related to: hypotension, bronchodilation, muscle relaxation, conjunctival injection, and decreased gastrointestinal motility. At the same point, for some people, those side effects could actually become a treatment. **That's up to you and your healthcare provider to determine.**

Cannabinoids are stored in 'adipose tissue' (body fat) and excreted at a very low rate. Researcher has shown a half-life 1–3 days. So even abruptly stopping use is not associated with any withdrawal symptoms. Because there are no rapid declines in plasma concentrations, there is no abrupt withdrawal symptoms or severe drug cravings. In general, THC can last in the adipose tissue, and blood stream, for up to 45 days from last use.

At the same time, users of cannabis need to understand that **cannabis plants are known 'soil remediates.' That means that they are toxin sponges**, and will suck up any and all toxins in the soil they are grown in, including any chemicals used to fertilize, as well as any pesticides or herbicides used. **Cannabis (including hemp) 'cleans' the soil,** and it's great at doing just that. Therefore, it's also important to know where the cannabis-based products is actually grown, if you're using them, because there are many countries with water we don't want to drink that leech toxins into the plant (sap and oil). As well as the potential for unaware growers using chemicals irresponsibly. Clean soil, awareness to the growing conditions, use of fertilizers, pesticides, herbicides, and responsible manufacturing are vital to safe product.

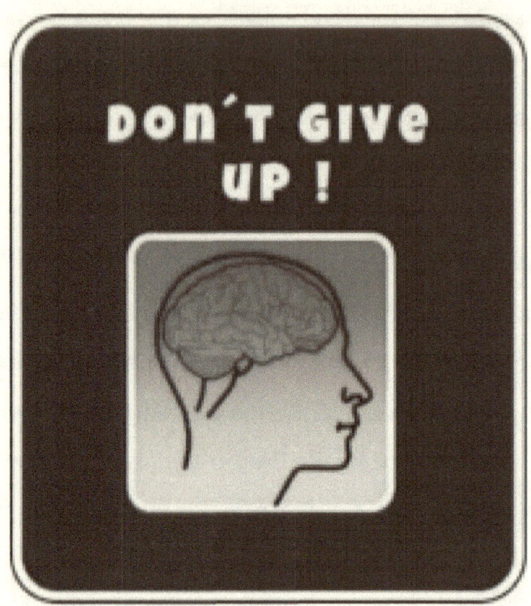

When used responsibly, and manufactured with awareness, at doses under 300mg a day for people with Parkinson's, under 600mg for most others, it seems to be safe… based on multiple safety studies done over the last 40+ years. However, the majority of scientific studies that have proven some health benefits include MORE THAN JUST CBD. It is just one of the components in nature's formula.

To date, there has yet to be any (even one) reported case of 'over dose' (even from higher levels of use) from either marijuana or CBD, but there have been thousands of reported over dose and serious side effects cases from the synthetic and FAKE STUFF!

1986, I.J.N., (International Journal of Neuroscience), published other studies. Their results: oral doses, ranging from 100 to 600 mg per day of cannabidiol were given to five patients with pre-existing dystonic movement disorders. In addition to recording specific benefits to those people. The study uncovered mild side effects with doses of 600mg of CBD and higher. They appeared to cause things like: hypotension, dry mouth, psychomotor slowing, lightheadedness, and sedation. During the study 2 patients with Parkinson's given CBD Oil, to quell their shakiness, **in doses over 300 mg per day seemed to actually experience AGGRAVATED** symptoms. Yet in 2014 a separate paper described how CBD significantly improves the lives of those with Parkinson's disease, so the verdict is still out on how much may (or may not) help those with Parkinson's. It's entirely possible it's based on a variety of other factors, such as diet, supplementation, age, weight, severity of the problem, location, exercise, genetics, etc. At this point, I would endeavor to keep the dose under 300mg per day if Parkinson's is an issue.

2011, ARITCLE ON MEDICINAL GENOMICS, stated that Grapefruit and CBD have a similar effect on P450, a key liver enzyme that metabolizes some drugs in the human body, particularly hepatic drugs. When large doses of CBD were taken it seems to inhibit the metabolizing properties of P450, which temporarily neutralized medicinal effects. It is also believed that this is also the reason the effects of THC are counteracted when large doses of CBD Oil are ingested. Again, caution is given if your issue requires P450.

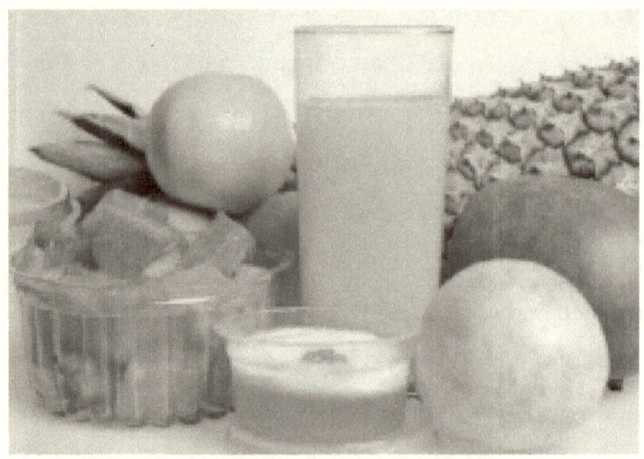

2018, SERIOUS WARNING: there were 51 reports of OVERDOSE in Utah, another 60 cases in North Carolina. However, all cases were linked to a product labeled "CBD" "K2" or "YOLO," and a variety of other names, usually coming straight from China. These products did NOT really or honestly CONTAIN any Cannabinol (no actual CBD Oil), but instead synthetic chemicals designed to 'create a HIGH' – like marijuana, rather than heal, help, or quell any symptoms. These fake products are sometimes ignorantly sold in vape shops, head shops, even small corner stores, and on the streets, or through some schools.

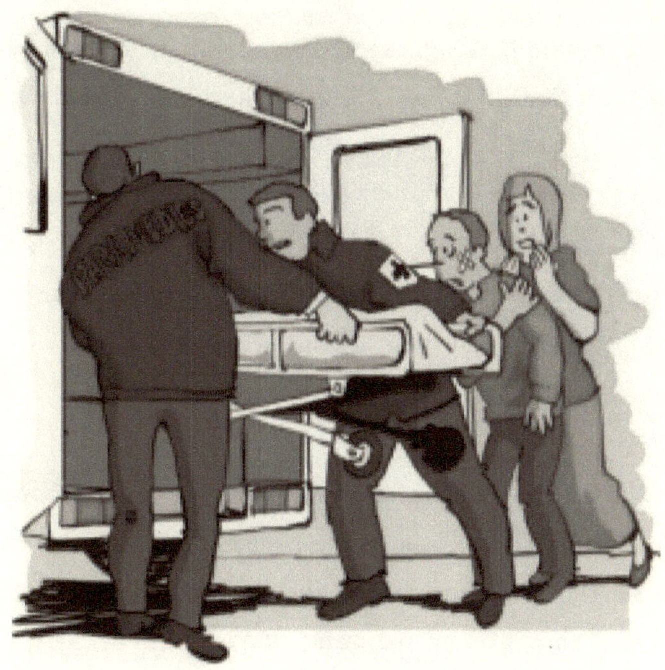

YOLO is a brand that used a synthetic substance called: 4-cyano CUMYL BUTINACA, but other chemicals found in some of the products were one of many synthetic cannabinoids, with cryptic ingredient names such as

- AB-CHMINACA,
- AB-FUBINACA.
- AB-PINACA
- AKB4,
- AM-2201 UR-144,
- Cannabicyclohexanol
- JWH-018,
- JWH-073,
- JWH-200,
- XLR-11,

Even the prescription drug, **phenazapam**, has been found in some of the fake or synthetic CBD products people selling them claimed were 'legal.'

The most popular brands sold today are Spice and K2, but the product 'Spice' has been reportedly sold 'private label,' under more than 600 different names, the most popular being: Mojo, Scooby Snax, Black Mamba, Spike, Annihilation, synthetic cannabis, fake pot, synthetic marijuana, legal weed, and herbal incense.

BE AWARE! To date, more than 1,000 kids, ages 12 to 18, have reported serious side effects, with some being hospitalized, ALL were tracked back to the SYNTHETIC stuff, fake marijuana, tainted vape juice, or FAKE CBD Oil. Things like: altered mental status, actual seizures, dysphoria and confusion, loss of consciousness, severe hallucinations, and even suicide. It's often packaged in a plastic packet that looks like a condom wrapper, or is sold in liquid form in a small dropper bottle that looks like normal vape juice, often with blue raspberries or some 'berry' on the label.

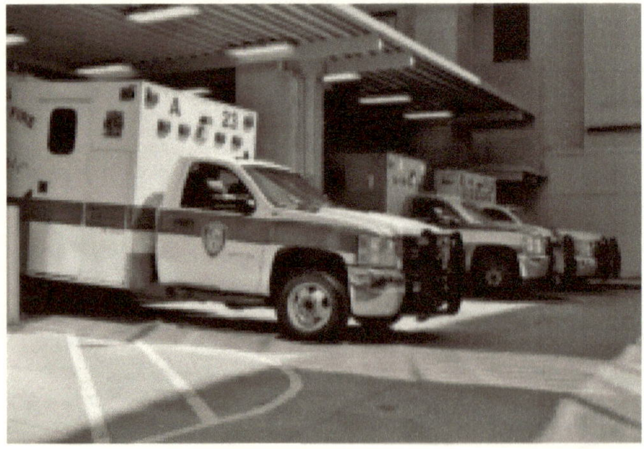

The problem is, unless you can see a COA you trust, people really don't know what they are really getting. READING THE LABELS helps. **For it to work right, medically, and consistently, it must be quantitative, consistent in both potency and type of chemical ingredients. If it's not, then the science can't be applied to OTHER products... that aren't the same.**

There are over a thousand (>1,000) reports of synthetic and herbal 'marijuana' and 'CBD' (none of which have anything to do with 'real' cannabis). Fake stuff causes problems, hallucinations, serious illness, and even death. Here are more common problem ingredients to be aware of:

- **Black Truffles** (Tuber melanosporum)
- **Cacao** (Theobroma cacao)
- **Chinese Rhododendron** - considered poisonous. Rhododendron

honey is known as "mad honey." Nevertheless, the leaves are used to make medicine.

- **Cotton Root** ~ (Aletris, Black Root, Canadian Hemp, Colombo, Cotton, Lavender Cotton Osha, Pleurisy Root, Queen's Delight, Sumbul) ~ Men using this herb for birth control should understand that it might cause irreversible sterility. There were cases of serious heart problems in many that use this herb.

- **Electric Daisy** (Acmella Oleracea)

- **Helichrysum** (Helichrysum italicum)

- **Japanese Liverwort** (Radula marginata)

- **Kava** (Piper methysticum, Kava-kava) - The use of kava for as little as one to three months has resulted in the need for liver transplants, and even death.

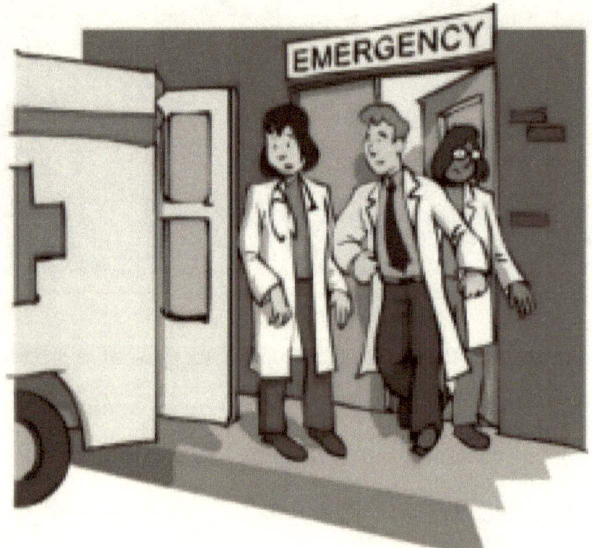

Each of those 'fake' products have different issues, concerns, and potential side effects, and **some of them are being 'sold as'** REAL! It's often children (high school to college age) that are reported to have issues with those products. They were blindly believing it is 'legal' and 'ok' because it's being sold over the counter in many stores. According to the CDC, the median time to onset of adverse reaction to these synthetics was usually within just minutes (often 1 to 10), though it does depend on exertion level, and the intact of other things that might increase or enhance their effects, such as alcohol or another drug. The duration of the adverse reaction lasted a median of 72 hours. The top adverse reactions reported were: altered mental status (82.4%), nausea or vomiting (49.0%), seizures or shaking (27.5%), loss of consciousness (25.5%) hallucinations (23.5%), and even SUICIDE! (They didn't disclose that number).

In liquid, usually a vape or droplet bottle, some of these synthetic products have a greater variety of chemicals… even within the same 'brand.' Scientists suspect a few brands may even contain traces of synthetic psychedelics such as 2C-P. In 2008, an analysis by the German government showed that some products contained almost none of herbs actually listed as ingredients on the packaging. When it comes to any 'synthetic' or 'herbal' remedies, it's always BUYER BEWARE!

The age group most often suffering is 12 to 18… too young to know any better. Unless are taught the very real world dangers and concerns, before temptation gives into opportunity, or peer pressure, ignorance will continue to be a problem. They need to be taught to QUESTION, to know what they are taking (and eating), and to THINK about the consequences of their own actions and choices.

Parents, babysitters, and even teachers have reported children they suspected, because of obvious reasons (such as seizures or passing out), to subtle changes in behavior (lethargic, staring off abnormally, lack of pupil response, attitude chances, etc.). They suspected the child might have 'gotten into,' or otherwise used, some type of drug; potentially having an adverse reaction. Rather than take any chances, or increase liability, they called in their concern – or authorities were notified.

Sometimes the child took whatever 'by accident,' edibles they didn't know contained drugs. Sometimes it was because of something a friend gave them (some knew 'it' contained or was drugs, some didn't). There were also reports of ingestion due to peer pressure, trying to either fit in, as well as an attempt to harm themselves.

When it's turned out to be JUST a cannabis product (usually some edibles, like brownies or gummies), the medical staff are generally able to relax, knowing **'pure cannabis' has never (yet) been the cause of an overdose death** for any person. **To date, neither THC or CBD have proven to be fatal or dangerous,** under the normal standards of 'overdose' and 'drug dangers' at levels upwards of an ounce per kilogram of body weight.

In 1973, scientists writing for the journal Toxicology and Applied Pharmacology noted "In dogs and monkeys, single oral doses of Δ9-THC and Δ8-THC between 3000 and 9000 mg/kg were nonlethal." Which was very clear, **3 to 9 grams THC per kilogram of body weight was non-lethal** to dogs and monkeys. (Other toxicity tests were later done on humans, finding similar results). It is impossible for the average human being to use, eat, smoke, or absorb enough chemicals normally found in cannabis to overdose). IT IS NOT PHYSICALLY POSSIBLE! 1 gram = 1000mg = 10,000ng ... so 3 grams = 3,000mg.

On the positive side, the responsible cannabis growers in the associations have agreed to start some 'standardized testing' for the raw – bulk cannabis product. It's a requirement in most of the 'legal' states: "a significant new compliance regime requiring each 10-pound lot [of marijuana or hemp] to be tested for potency, microbial contamination and pesticide residues by a licensed, accredited laboratory." [prior to processing] The goal is self-protection, and to distinguish themselves from the backyard growers that aren't doing the volume, and can't afford the testing (which isn't cheap).

According to Johnathan Rubin, CEO of Cannabis Benchmarks, there are additional bureaucratic compliance, licensing, and testing requirements to consider in California. [It's frankly unclear what happens to the tested product, or how the bulk is selected, or whether it includes buds and flowers, which are higher in THC levels, or just stems and leaves, or seeds, which aren't as high, to purposefully test lower. **It's quite evident that many companies don't appear eager to test finished product,** but instead quote the 'raw material' test maximum levels, tests the growers did, to remain in compliance for their Government Approved 'Hemp Pilot Program']

MEDICAL USE CAN BE IMPORTANT

In **1998, THE BRITISH GOVERNMENT LICENSED A COMPANY TO GROW CANNABIS**, and develop a precise and consistent extract for use in clinical trials. England knew that Queen Victoria used cannabis for menstrual cramps, and other ailments, in the 19th century; and saw it used enough throughout the centuries to know it was safe and beneficial.

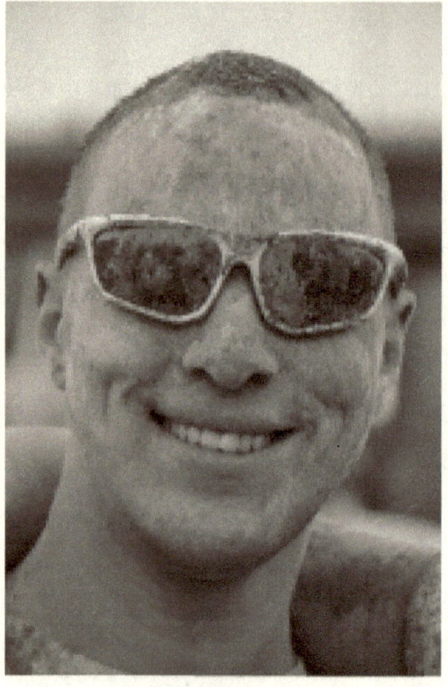

On October 17th 2018 Canada made all cannabis products legal, for medical AND recreational use. Uruguay legalized it all in 2017, after years of planning (cough, how the government could regulate and profit from the regulation and sales of it).

The oils had mostly been forgotten, or kept buried as some little secret, until the 'push' for a 'smoke-less' and 'legal by-pass' was needed. Then CBD production and scientific research really stepped up as a means to basically 'have the cake and eat it too' for the medical world.

It was developed to eliminate the need to 'smoke' (in light of the world's rejection of 'smoking' and equation of smoking to lung cancer, as well as the reality that no one could expect a child to 'start smoking' to get their 'medication'), and also to reduce the THC levels (the markers most governments use to test for marijuana use) while increasing the medicinal value and benefits.

There are also indications that low doses (100 to 300mg a day) of CBD Oil has helped some of those suffering from Parkinson's, BUT doses above 300mg per day can actually make the symptoms and challenges worse.

There are finally some acknowledgements, by government agencies, that **CBD+THC (the combination) can even help certain types of cancer.** The science that supported that is why the FDA APPROVED DRONABINOL AND NABILONE, for the treatment of certain 'cancer-related side effects.'

The reality of science seems extremely promising. However, as a company, our primary focus is on NUTRITION: vitamins, minerals, and nutrients natural to the body, not herbs or botanicals. So any evaluation of the marijuana, THC, or CBD science has nothing to do with our company, until or unless it became 100% legal under both Federal and

State Laws. Even then, we'd likely avoid selling it.

AUGUST 1, 2018, FIRST CANADIAN PEDIATRIC study of mixed THC/CBD cannabis oil for children with drug-resistant epilepsy shows promise, and is worth watching. October 17th 2018, all cannabis was decriminalized in Canada.

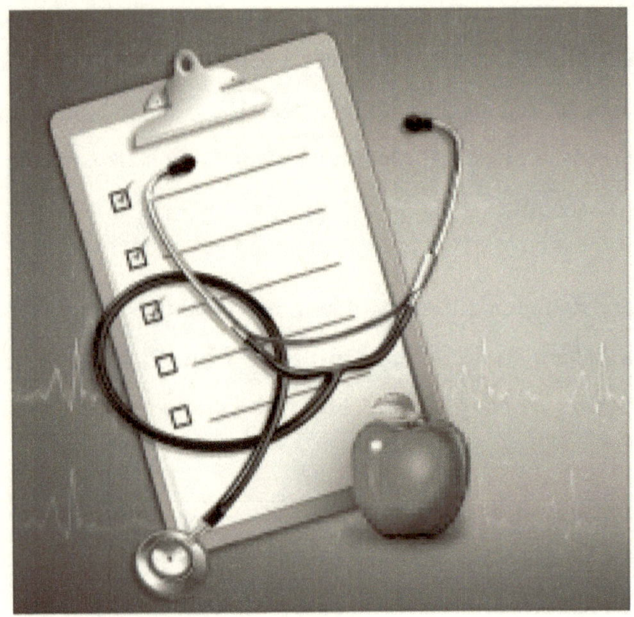

Page Intentionally Left Blank for Your Own Notes:

FIGURING THE DOSING (POTENCY)

"One Eye Dropper of CBD per day" (1 ml) seems to be what most CBD sales people say, and labels promote. Which means a 30ml bottle is designed to last a month, at just one dropper full a day. Remember, most treatments, require splitting the dose into two or three times a day. However, **we've seen potencies fluctuate from less than 1mg per ml, to as much as 600mg per dose**, coming out of exactly the same 'looking' bottle. That is a huge variance, and the dose would absolutely matter a great deal if you are actually trying to treat something.

The math, matters. Any company that promotes a 'one size fits all' type of dosage recommendation really shouldn't be trusted, ever! They really don't understand the science, or the reality that individual factors, like weight, age, severity, precise problem, body chemistry, other medications and treatments, and type of condition all matter. **There really is no 'fits all' single dose.**

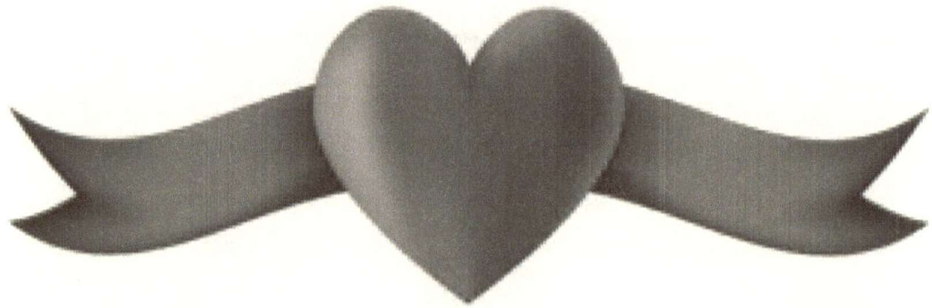

In general, the dose considered 'normal' and 'safe' for most otherwise healthy and normal people, is 1-6mg of CBD for every 10 pounds of body weight, based on the pain level; assuming epilepsy, cancer, or nervous disorders aren't involved. So, the average 160lb person, without severe or serious health issues, would use approximately 16 to 96mg per day. The easiest way to calculate 'strength' is **[Total actual mg's of CBD in Bottle] ÷ [Number of Milliliters in Bottle] = mg per ml (which is usually one normal full dropper)**.

Ideally, look for products that PROPORTITIONALLY offer both THC and CBD, rather than false claims of 'zero' THC. Look at the science for what you are attempting to treat, help, prevent, or cure… TALK WITH YOUR HEALTHCARE PROVIDER… and remember, **nearly all proactive positive and beneficial science shows a ratio of CBD and THC (from 1:1, to 1:6)**. And some, certain cancer cells, have actually responded negatively to too much THC. So, awareness of the actual science, and that professional opinion, is even more important.

Another factor is tolerance. Most people start at the lower dosage, and increase a little each week, if the pain or problem doesn't significantly reduce after a few days. A person should be careful, and monitor how their individual body deals with things. Start small and increase GRADUALLY, as needed.

If you have any serious medical condition or concern, you should absolutely consult your physician. There are not, currently, a whole lot of doctors that really know about CBD Oil, the differences or dosage, the doctors generally understand the dosage math, and your individual body history.

Like most drugs, there is an issue of the 'First-pass elimination.' As Drs. Pond and Tozer, explain, "[It] takes place when a drug is metabolized between its site of administration and the site of sampling for measurement of drug concentration. Clinically, first-pass metabolism is important when the fraction of the dose administered that escapes metabolism is small and variable. The liver is usually assumed to be the major site of first-pass metabolism of a drug administered orally, but other potential sites are the gastrointestinal tract, blood, vascular endothelium, lungs, and the arm from which venous samples are taken. Bioavailability, defined as the ratio of the areas under the blood concentration-time curves, after extra- and intravascular drug administration (corrected for dosage if necessary), is often used as a measure of the extent of first-pass metabolism."

Next, **consider the actual measuring, for accurate dosing**. The average eye dropper is 1 ml when filled with an average full squeeze, but do you really know how many milligrams you're getting in that dropper? There are some pre-measured pills or gel caps, which are easy and consistent.

The 'best' way to use CBD Oil is nearly as variable as how do you like your coffee. Many claim allowing the oil to 'sit' under your tongue for 30 to 90 seconds before swallowing is best; because the smallest molecules can be absorbed, sublingually. The next highest absorption is reported to be rectally (for the oil), though we've seen little actual science proving CBD is more bio-available that way, such studies have been done with other chemicals… and proven true. Both methods by-pass the digestive tract, eliminating any extra breaking down, or apart, the chemicals.

Those sales people that claim 'it is all the same' – whether you put it under your tongue, use it rectally, put it in a cold drink, over hot food, in a cigarette, or vaporizer… clearly they do not understand just how science works, or how wrong they are. The absorption is absolutely not the same. Really, can you trust the advice from people that don't understand the differences? That believe there is a 'one size fits all' dose? Don't know which OTHER cannabinoids are actually IN their product? Or that claim there is 'zero' THC???

Most CBD products cannot honestly offer any proof of bioavailability, but there are sure a bunch of them that will claim it. Eating some fat or oil, nuts or full-fat yogurt, will improve absorption when CBD is eaten. Cannabinoids love fat, and are readily taken up by the small intestine, when they make it that far. The majority of CBD products do not offer any bioavailability optimization (most of those manufacturer's don't even know what they means).

They are just 'panning for gold' and 'striking while the iron is hot' – pushing a product they falsely claim is legal in all 50 states, under all circumstances, that can cures a zillion problems (at least according to them, and their marketing). The reality is that there is **a mountain of marketing claims pushing a grain of sand product** in most cases. Actual science – using different products and higher level of ingredients, often including THC and other key cannabinoids, produced actual results that all these other companies are claiming their product is capable of, without any actual science on their product… or matching COA showing they have all the right ingredients, at the right levels..

Understand, in general, it has been stated that 'smoking' offers a bioavailability of 25%, meaning 100mg in a cigarette would become approximately 25mg 'to the body.' It's unknown what the circumstances were for that calculation, or the exact math for conversion in a vaporizer. Obviously, how a person inhales, how long they hold the smoke, and the amount of heat used to produce the vapor will all be variances that impact what actually makes it into the body.

Soft gels have a lower bio-availability, and edibles even less bioavailability for CBD; because of the fluctuation of manufacturing and acids in the digestive tract.

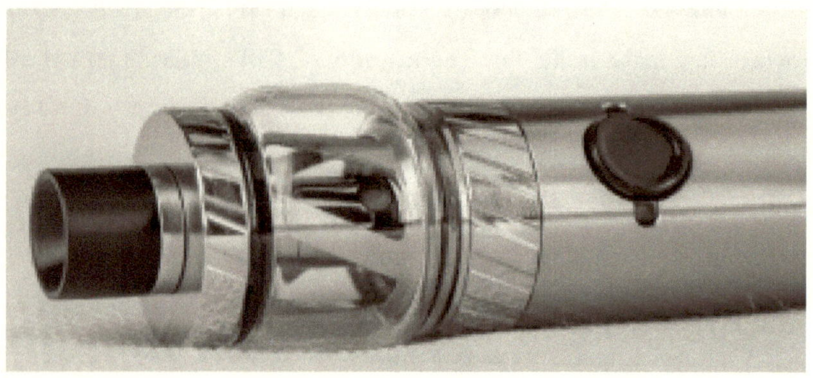

It is nearly impossible to properly measure your dose in a vaporizer. The variables are exponential, based on heat of the coils, length of the draw, starting mg, number of inhales per day, depth of the inhale (mouth vs full lungs), and other factors.

With vaping, the math is more challenging, because you need to keep count of how much you put in the tank, how many 'draws' it takes before you need to refill, and how many times a day you actually refill... and frankly, whether you inhale into the lungs, and hold it in. All variables that impact the math, and usually least absorption.

Be aware of storage issues, and requirements. Unless the packaging or manufacturer tells you otherwise, you should refrigerate after opening!

Page Left Intentionally Blank for Your Notes:

COMMONLY STUDIED CANNABINOIDS:

Before we jump to the meat, we need to understand, contrary to what hundreds of millions of people were taught just a few years ago, Pluto is no longer considered a 'planet' in our solar system, but now a 'dwarf planet' (like the other 'new' dwarf plants found, thanks to some space exploration: Ceres, Eris, Haumea, Makemake, and Planet x).

The point is: **Science evolves.** But, so does marketing, advertising, and the illusions used to give false hope and over generalized claims. The illusion of unscrupulous marketing is often to use some grains of truth to push an unrelated product. It's pushed by those without either knowledge or ethics, willing to twist facts, attempting to claim it's 'all the same' and 'just like,' when they know it really isn't, because they don't really care about other people's lives.

New things are learned, clarified, reclassified, found, discovered, and even invented or created each year. Some things are repurposed, new things invented, some really do evolve. However, one should be careful, and aware.

There is a considerable variance in cannabis plants, from grower to grower, even harvest to harvest (with the same grower). "There is NOT a reproducibly consistent chemical profile with predictable or even consistent clinical effects." They imply that cannabis is not like Beefsteak Tomato's, Iceberg Lettuce, peanuts, or a Douglas Fir tree – which are pretty much the same around the world, with a +/- x% difference in micro nutrients because of soil or fertilizer differences, pesticide choices, or other micro factors.

However, there is a group that jumps out claiming all cannabis should be the same, and perfectly consistent. But it isn't. No two plants are exactly the same, nor are the flowers, leaves, stems, or seeds from the same plant even the same; just like no two people are exactly the same; even identical twins have subtle differences. Unless you have special tools, training, and experience, it is nearly impossible for the average person to even visually tell if a diamond is real or not. Especially with the man-made versions now able to 'cut glass' and resist chipping.

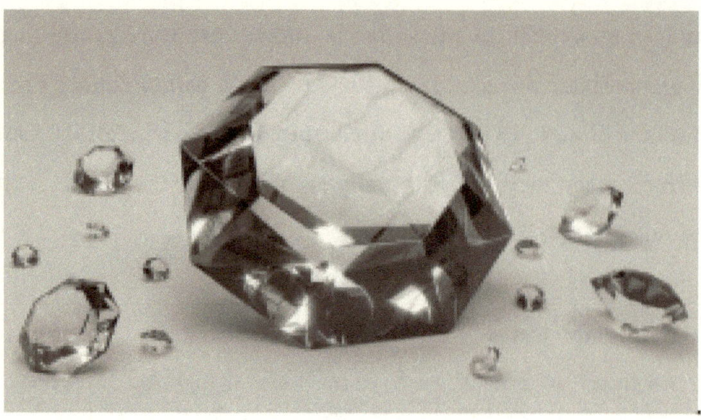

Cannabis strains have been almost as varied as the female dog that breeds whatever, so there is little actual predictability from litter to litter, with vastly different constituents. Worse, there are over 500 different components making up the average cannabis plant, and only 113 have officially been named and somewhat tracked for cause and effect. That inconsistency and unpredictability is part of the reason the government claims 'cannabis' (marijuana, weed, pot, etc.) is illegal... and needs to be a controlled substance. Those are just well rehearsed talking points and excuses, with many years of refinement.

Some people in power know different, but have benefitted from the 'War on Drugs.' Some have bothered to look through some of the science, many know marijuana isn't what the 'death drug' the government has historically claimed it to be. The real reason it is illegal, and a 'controlled substance' is ultimately control… and money. (more on that later).

With legalized cannabis, like in Canada & Uruguay, the general public can grow, exchange, trade, barter with, and use cannabis products. Those wanting to be in charge doesn't have much control, or profit from it, and those things are what concerns them. It is easier to selectively enforce laws, especially since none are exactly the same.

THE ELEVEN SYSTEMS IN THE HUMAN BODY:

1. Circulatory/Vascular – blood, arteries and veins,

2. Digestive – eating to pooping, nutrient absorption,

3. Endocrine – glands and hormones,

4. Integumentary – skin, hair, nails,

5. Lymphatic / Immune – lymph nods, filtration, marrow

6. Muscular – allows movement of the body

7. Nervous – transmits signals from body to brain, pleasure and pain

8. Respiratory – breathing (gas exchange in the body via lungs)

9. Reproductive – procreation (off spring, continuation of species)

10. Skeletal – 206 bones, also ligaments, tendons, and cartilage, gives shape to the body, allowing movement, strength, and support of body

11. Urinary/renal - eliminate waste from the body, regulates blood volume and blood pressure, control levels of electrolytes and metabolites, regulate blood pH, and helps clean the blood.

All those systems make up the human body (and that of all mammals). However, in the late 1990's, some medical researchers claimed to find a 12th system. They published their findings in a 2002 peer reviewed journal; shaking up much of the medical field.

However, it is still not completely accepted by 100% of the medical profession. Nearly all research scientists, especially those working with cancer and neurological systems, and most all of those doctors working with medical cannabis agree that it is **the 12th SYSTEM in mammal's bodies.**

Since the initial findings, most medical research scientists are claiming that system is the ENDOCANNABINOID SYSTEM (ECS), which all vertebrates and invertebrates have since been proven to have. That system has a direct impact on the immune system, pain receptors, and nervous system. It is considered the most important system for MAINTAINING HEALTH by many researchers.

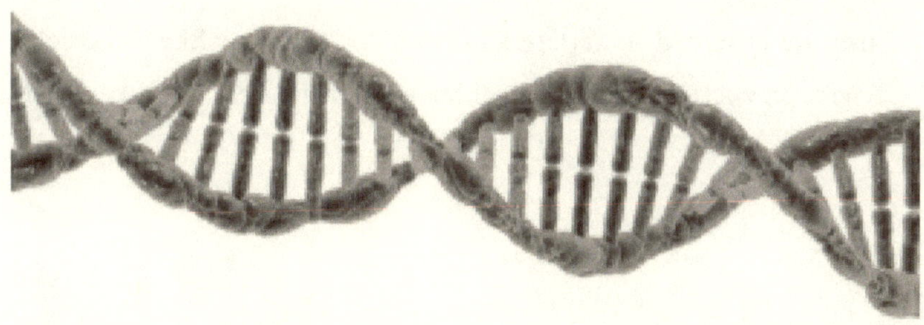

The endocannabinoids created and used in the mammals body are vital, because they help regulate the dopamine (a neurotransmitter that helps control the brain's reward and pleasure center); and it also helps regulate movement and emotional responses. Dopamine enables us to not only see specific rewards, through our senses and mind, but to actually take action to move toward those perceived rewards.

Contrary to some marketing claims, science has shown that there really is no THC actually 'made by' the human body. 'Endocannabinoids' are not the same as THC (tetrahydrocannabinol)!

There are 'Endocannabinoids'... found in every mammal's body. These chemicals are made naturally by the body, just like insulin, adrenalin, dopamine, serotonin, and so many other amino acids, and enzymes. They are naturally occurring substances, expected and normal in every body.

Contrary to rumors in the 90's, endocannabinoids are not the same as THC, and (again) THC is not 'made by' or from, anything 'naturally found in' the human body. Yes, there are cannabinoids in the body, but they are different! As different as red blood cells vs white blood cells, with very different purposes, although both are vital components of 'blood.'

Page Intentionally Left Blank for Your Own Notes:

THREE TYPES OF CANNABINOIDS:

- **ENDOCANNABINOIDS** (found naturally, in the body)
- **PHYTOCANNABINOIDS** (found in plants)
- **SYNTHETIC CANNABINOIDS** (man-made or even fake)

CBD, like THC, interacts primarily with the brain neurons, which are specialized cells in your central nervous system (the brain and spinal cord) that transmits and interprets all nerve impulses, which is the pathway and control center for all five senses... plus pain, thought, emotions. Both voluntary and involuntary actions.

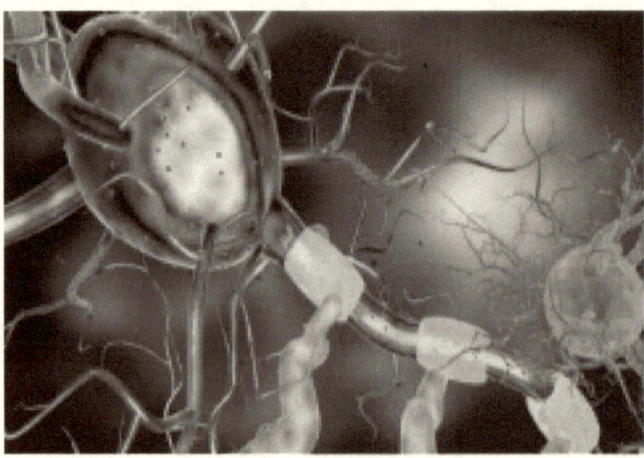

Assistant Professor at the Boston University School of Social Work, Christopher P. Salas-Wright, said the 'number of credible studies already provide compelling evidence that marijuana (and CBD Oil) use has increased meaningfully among adults in general, middle-aged and older adults in particular, over the last 10 to 15 years."

Late 2017, the World Health Organization (WHO) came out publicly, stating that cannabidiol (CBD), a component in medical marijuana, does NOT HAVE A RISK for abuse, and is not 'addictive' like its counterpart, THC (another component in cannabis).

The first cannabinoid-like chemicals naturally found in the human body to be discovered was Anandamide, in the 1990's. Repeated and verified, then officially mentioned in a peer reviewed medical journal in 2002. The fatty acid, also known as AEA, is 'a neurotransmitter derived from non-oxidative metabolism of eicosatetraenoic acid (ETA).' Anandamide acts on both the CB-1 and CB-2 receptors, modulating both the central and peripheral nervous system, respectively.

The right amount of quality CBD Oil can activate receptors in the brain that THC can't: such as, the adenosine, serotonin, and vanilloid receptor.

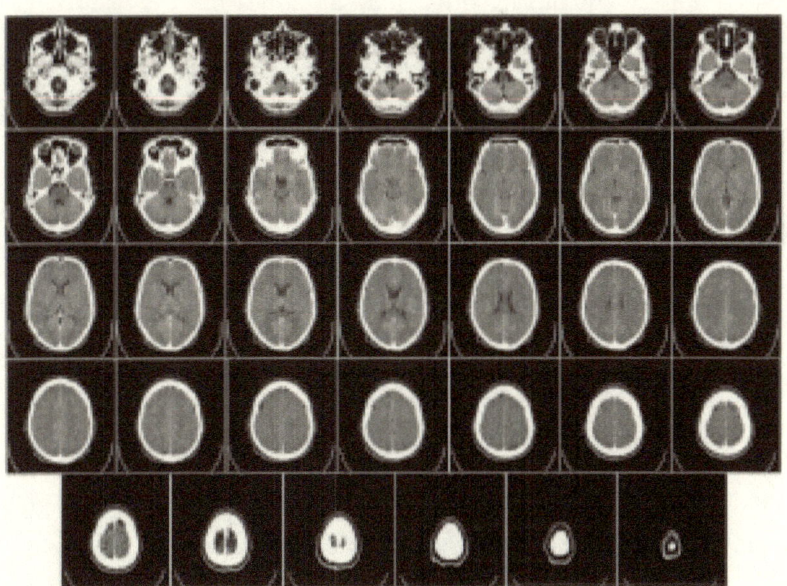

When introduced into the body, here's what those specific receptors do:

- **CB1 AND CB2** - are Class A (rhodopsin family) G-protein-coupled receptors (GPCRs), naturally occurring within mammals bodies, they impact (and effect) the dopamine receptors. Science has shown these receptors regulate and directly impact learning, coordination, sleep, pain, and the immune system.

  - The **ADENOSINE** receptor - resultant brain activity reduces anxiety.
  - The **SEROTONIN** receptor - reduces depression, alters blood sugar levels, limits nausea, and a whole host of other neurological effects.
  - The **VANILLOID** receptor - limits the 'feeling' of pain and inflammation, masking symptoms.

Studies have proven that cannabidiol does NOT affect short term memory loss; however, THC does.

For those in the over 50 crowd, which might have tried marijuana in the 60's through 80's, **it's important to understand that the stuff out there today is NOT THE SAME!** In fact, studies, such as those done by Goulle and Guerbet, have shown that the THC level has risen by at least a factor of 4, from 4% to 16%, over the last 20 years [speculating that there was another rise in potency in the 20 to 30 years prior to that, as strains were cultivated for increased potency, higher yield, and different 'taste' and smells].

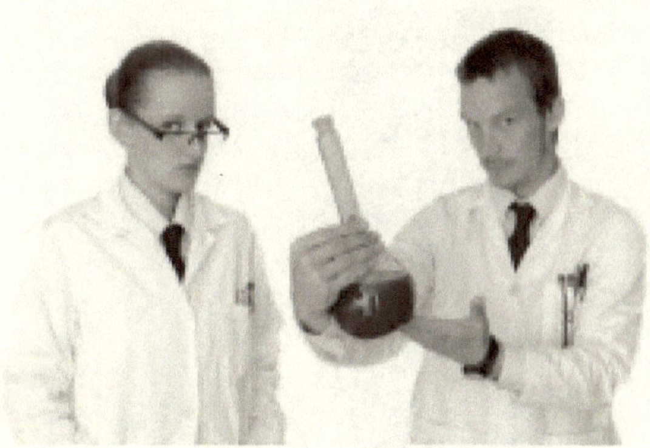

Their research showed that, "This increase [in potency] has important implications not only for the pharmacokinetics, but also for the pharmacology of THC.

The bioavailability of THC, in smoked cannabis, is about 25%. In a cigarette (or 'joint') containing just 3.55% of THC, a peak plasma level of about 160ng/mL occurs approximately 10 min after inhalation. ('ng' is 'nanograms' per 'ml' (milliliter)).

THC is quickly cleared from plasma, in a multiphasic manner, and is widely distributed to tissues; which leads to pharmacologic effects felt in the body (cough, realization of the impact starting in THE BRAIN).

Body fat is a long-term storage site; so it can be retained longer in a person that is over weight than someone without as much extra fat (for unintended storage). This particular pharmacokinetic behavior found in that study explains the lack of correlation between the THC blood level and clinical effects, contrary to ethanol. Another words, intoxication and impairment isn't as clear, obvious, or easy to test with marijuana as it is alcohol.

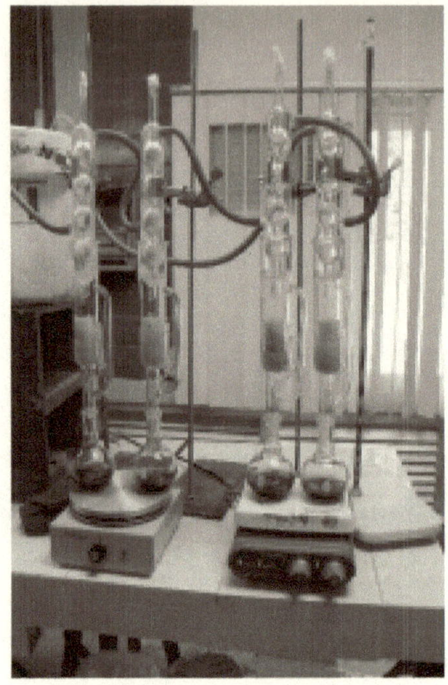

The list below are just some of the MOST COMMONLY STUDIED cannabinoids found in cannabis plants. There are over 113 specifically identified, and nearly 500 isolated cannabinoids. Some speculate they are as widely different as petroleum products, from the plastic used for the gasoline container to rocket fuel, with assorted levels, uses, and types in between. However, what most people may not realize is that the human body actually produces its own 'cannabinoids,' in the endogenous cannabinoid system (ECS).

These are natural equivalents similar to the compounds found in the cannabis plant, such as CBD (cannabidiol). **Here are 34 of the most studied cannabinoids:**

- CBC - cannabichromene
- CBC-C5 - Cannabichromene
- CBCA - cannabichromenate
- CBCA-C5A - Cannabichromenic acid A
- CBCV-C3 - Cannabichromevarin
- CBCVA - Cannabichromevarinic acid
- CBCVA-C3A - Cannabichromevarinic acid A

- CBD - Cannabidiol
- CBD-C1 - Cannabidiorcol
- CBD-C4 - Cannabidiol-C4
- CBD-C5 – cannabidiol C5
- CBDA - cannabidolic acid
- CBDA-C5 - cannabidiolic acid C5
- CBDM-C5 - Cannabidiol momomethyl ether
- CBDV - cannabidivarin
- CBDVA- C3 - cannabidivarinic acid C3
- CBDV-C3 -Cannabidivarin

- CBG - cannabigerol
- CBGA - cannabigerolic acid
- CBGA-C3A - Cannabigerolic acid A –C3
- CBGA-C5A - Cannabinerolic acid A – C5
- CBGAM-C5A - Cannabigerolic acid A monomethyl ether – C5

- CBG-C5 – Cannabigerol – C5
- CBGM-C5A - Cannabigerolmonomethyl ether – C5
- CBGVA-C5A - Cannabigerovarinic acid A – C5
- CBGV-C – Cannabigerovarin

- CBL - cannabicyclol
- CBLA – cannabicyclol acid

- CBN - cannabinol
- CBND-C3 – cannabinodivarin – C3
- CBND-C5 - cannabinodiol – C5

- CBT - cannabicitran

Also important, when any cannabinoid acids are heated (i.e., smoked, or heat processed, vaped, or baked) they lose the "A" (acid) part, and turn into neutral (rather than remain acidic). CBN is formed by degradation and oxidization of THC

Again, **tetrahydrocannabinol (THC) is NOT 'natural to' or 'made by' the human body.** The 'runners high,' which has been historically attributed to endorphins (the body's self-produced opiates) have been found to actually be endocannabinoids, as demonstrated in a 2015 study done at the University of Oxford, UK. They are not THC, but are a cannabinol that impacts the dopamine's. Cannabinols are NATURALLY FOUND IN EVERY mammal's body, including human beings, and are most prevalently found in the brain and spinal column.

If you test positive for THC it is because you smoked, breathed, ingested, or somehow took a product containing THC. There is NONE, zero, zilch naturally or normally found in the human body. (Contrary to rumors and some claims) The 'cannabinoids' made by the body are natural, normal, and do not contain, and are not, the same as THC.

Most cannabinoids will not cause any intoxicating effect, or 'get you high.' THC is the only known cannabinoid that can for sure do that to most mammals, including most all human beings! However, **science has shown that the presence of the other cannabinoids can absolutely impact HOW THC affects a body, because those cannabinoids influence how THC interacts with the receptors in the endocannabinoid system (ECS) within the body of mammals.**

In nature, all plants are organic, but not everything organic is good, safe, or beneficial to a mammals body. If you doubt me, consider what hemlock does, or sumac, or the array of other 'all natural' poisons that are organic.

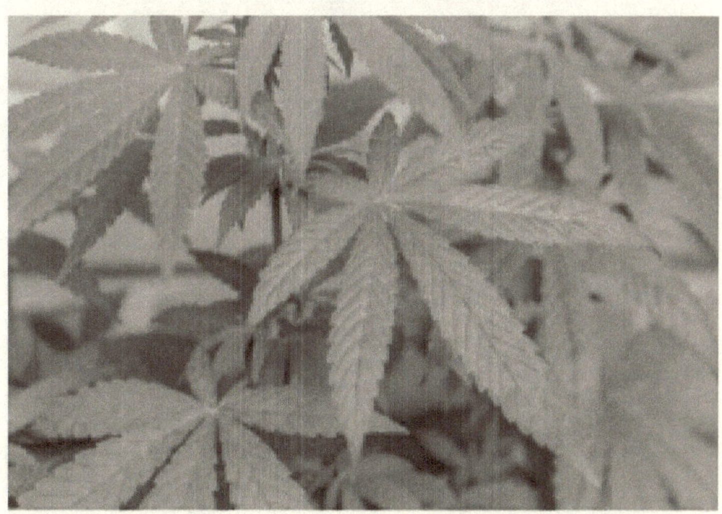

With that said, **I have NOT been able to find even one report of an over dose of marijuana THC**, though there were some reports of too much CBD Oil causing issues in Parkinson's patients, and at least one study that showed too much THC could INCREASE the growth of at least one type of cancer cell (while many studies show killing, slowing, or eliminating growth of OTHER types of cancer cells)… and no seeming impact on other types. Hopefully you'll never have to find out, or have a variety is CAN HELP. Please… before trying to self-medicate – TALK WITH YOUR HEALTH CARE PROVIDER, and a real doctor that has been studying the type of cancer in question.

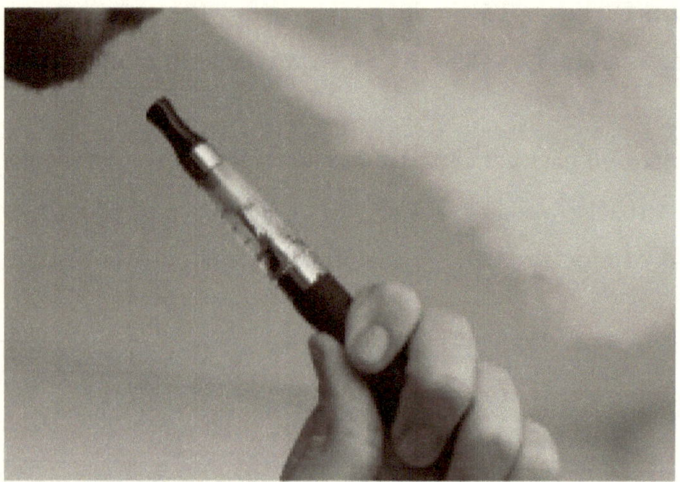

There are over 25,000 abstracts (science articles and studies) on cannabis, THC and CBDs, for medicinal use… and safety. Yet, fewer than 500 found on alcohol, and only a handful on vaping (none about vaping CBD oils as of early 2019). Wrap your head around those numbers.

Page Intentionally Left Blank for Your Own Notes:

ARE HEMP & MARIJUANA THE SAME?

Short Answer: Nope, no more than a St. Bernard is the same as a Chihuahua, or either are the same as a wolf; however, they are all 'dogs,' in the family of 'canis.' Different 'species' in the same kingdom, phylum, class, order, and family.

Marijuana and hemp are two different species of plants <u>from same family</u>, the genus: Cannabis… and today, the federal laws specify 'cannabis.'

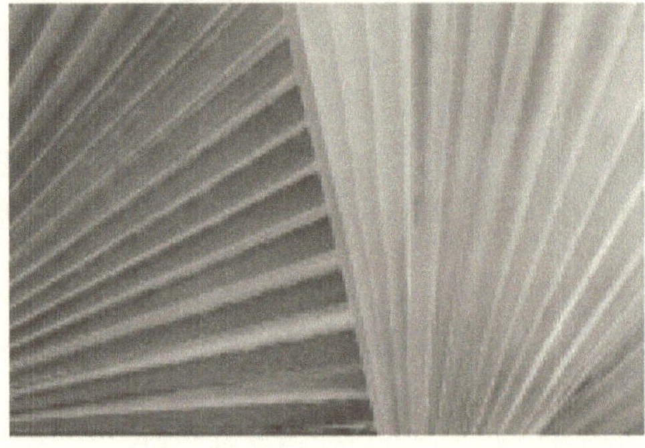

That's equivalent to saying they didn't ban 'wolves' – but ALL DOGS! When they detailed their Schedule I Controlled Substance Act Laws, "all cannabis – and derivatives of" were specifically banned. That technically and absolutely includes HEMP, at this time, which is also in the 'cannabis' species. Much like different types of horses, dogs, snakes, roses, or tomatoes... they each have small genetic variations, which can be significant. These slight genetic differences change what they do, how they do it, and create assorted other subtle to extreme differences, often far more complexity than just size, color, or taste variations.

The primary (known) difference is the level of THC naturally found in the stem, leaves, flowers, and buds. In general, Industrial Hemp has less than 0.3% (one third of one percent) of THC; whereas Marijuana can contain as much as 30% in the buds and flowers, upwards of 20% in the leaves, and up to 16% in the stems and seeds. Contrary to most of the marketing claims, **CBD cannot be extracted from hempseed**. This is key to figuring out just how much a sales person knows, or if the label is honest.

Also, some sales people have claimed that "legal CBD oil coverts to THC in the digestive tract" which is a complete joke, and scenically proven to be 100% false! The science relied up on, by Gaoni and Mechoulam (1968) was done in a similar fashion to that mentioned in Reefer Madness, and other propaganda information, in simulated highly unnatural settings, which had nothing to do with real-life human experience (or how it would actually work in a mammal's bodies).

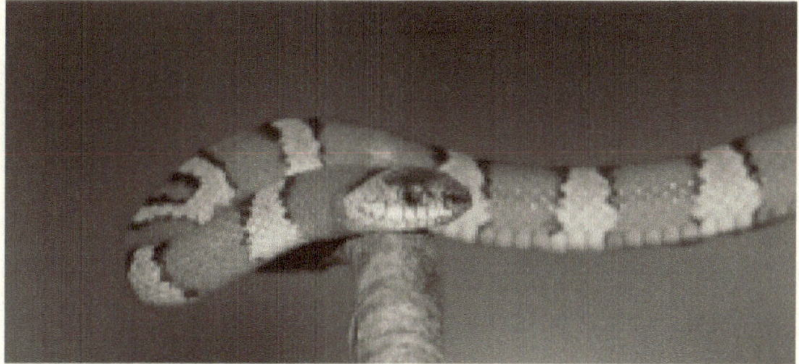

It's more difficult for the average person to tell the difference between marijuana and industrial hemp, than between a King snake and Coral snake, as there is no cute little saying to help people learn to differentiate them. "Red next to black, is a friend of Jack. Red next to yellow can kill a fellow." Problem solved, for if you come across one of the snakes. But it won't help you with cannabis.

It's also far more difficult than telling the difference between a rose and daisy, or clover… or even between a good wine and expensive wine. Either type of cannabis can be grown more quickly and easier than corn, tomato plants, or even the grass in your lawn; but it can also be as technically challenging as Orchids or champion Iris's or Roses, for those wanting to tweak genetics and play with cross breeding.

John Merrick et. Al. (2015) expressed concerns that such misinformation could skew public policy and regulatory decisions at a time when cannabinoid therapies are gaining favor. It's speculated that the 'rumor' was started by companies knowing their CBD product contained high levels of THC, in an attempt to shift their responsibility (or rather lack of) in honest advertising and lacking tests (or deceitful disclosures). Grotenhermen, et. Al (2107) proved that dosing up to 600mg of quality CBD oil does not cause THC-like effects, or skew test results for THC.

At the same time, there are studies that show very small amounts of THC are excreted in urine after the ingestion of some CBD products.

Typically, marijuana is grown, crossed, and genetically cultivated to have high amounts of tetrahydrocannabinol (THC), which is a psycho-active chemical compound that generally 'mellowed' people out over centuries, and reduced a variety of chronic pains… or gets them really 'high.' Whereas, Industrial Hemp came about by trying to purposefully reduce the amount of THC, so it might be legally grown without breaking the law.

The 'natural herb' that was made most popular during the 'hippy movement' of the 60's and 70's, and given infamy by the Cheech & Chong "Up In Smoke" series of movies is significantly different today. Cannabis has evolved, through horticultural magic, and genetic manipulation. It is not the same today as it was in the 60's or even the 70's, it is generally at least 400% stronger. The effects are often vastly different because of genetic tweaking, cross breeding with different strains, and more of a scientific genetic laboratory application that altered and improved the growing process. Their goals were as varied as increasing the THC potency, improving flavor, calming harshness, increasing growth rate, production volume, improving flavors, or some combinations thereof. In general, a plant can go from seed to harvest in as little as 3 months, under optimum conditions; though the strongest strains can take up wards of 6 to 9 months, usually with a 2 or 3 week 'curing' process.

In general, high THC absorption can lead to a peaceful euphoric feeling, to almost total paranoia; depending on the variety and the individual. To those wanting to 'get high' (wasted, stoned, mellow, etc), marijuana with THC is what they are looking for. It is the psychoactive chemical in cannabis plants that creates the reaction. CBD is not psychoactive, and won't get you 'high.'

THC has actually triggered panic attacks (and paranoia), because it impacts the neurotransmitters involved in the 'fight or flight' response (promoting FLIGHT, which is why so few 'stoners' and 'pot heads' got into fights in the 60's and 70's – during the 'peace & love' movement. CBD eases anxiety and is calming, but it's not that way 100% of the time. Some research has shown that a subset of people that have used high levels of THC experienced serious and debilitating anxiety, even paranoia.

In some, rare cases, it can trigger the onset of schizophrenia in those that seem to have a genetic predisposition to that disease. So, knowing the individual history and watching the levels of THC, is important.

Bottom line: they aren't all the same, the reality is they vary and are not even exactly the same from batch to batch, harvest to harvest.

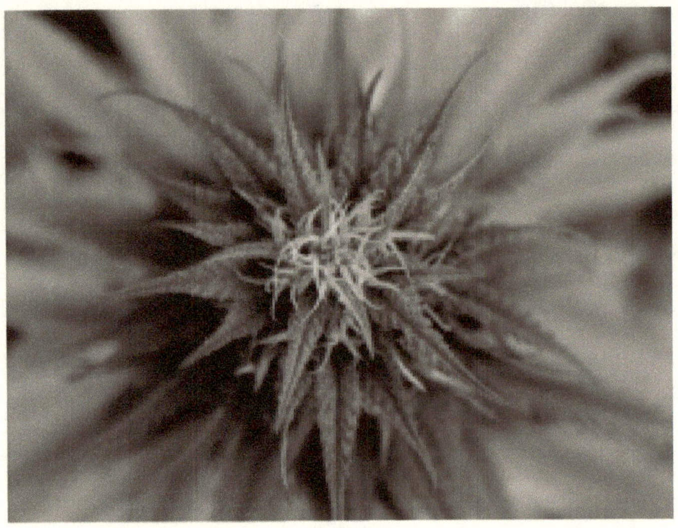

Hemp, on the other hand, is bred specifically to have trace amounts of THC, lowest possible amounts, less than 0.3% is the legal requirements for 'industrial grade' hemp. Certainly not enough to cause any psychoactive effect.

The end products from hemp have been historically used to make rope, paper, clothing, biofuel, plastic composites, construction materials, concrete, animal bedding, insulation, netting, canvas, cardboard, and so many other things all around the world.

The last five years, they have been squeezing the 'sap' out of the stems and leaves to make CBD Oil, much like Flax seed oil, Linseed oil, or other plant oils. Usually with the same type of processing.

Like bamboo, under the right conditions, cannabis is extremely fast and easy to grow. It is easy to care for, and has been proven to enrich the soil in which it grows, cleaning it from heavy metals and toxins, and adding good nutrients to the soil, all for other varieties of crops. Seriously, from seed to harvest in as little as 3 months.

TWO TYPES OF 'CHRONIC PAIN'

- **NEUROGENIC PAIN** –results from actual damage to the nerves
- **PSYCHOGENIC PAIN** – which is NOT due to a genetic malformation, past injury, disease, or visible sign of damage.

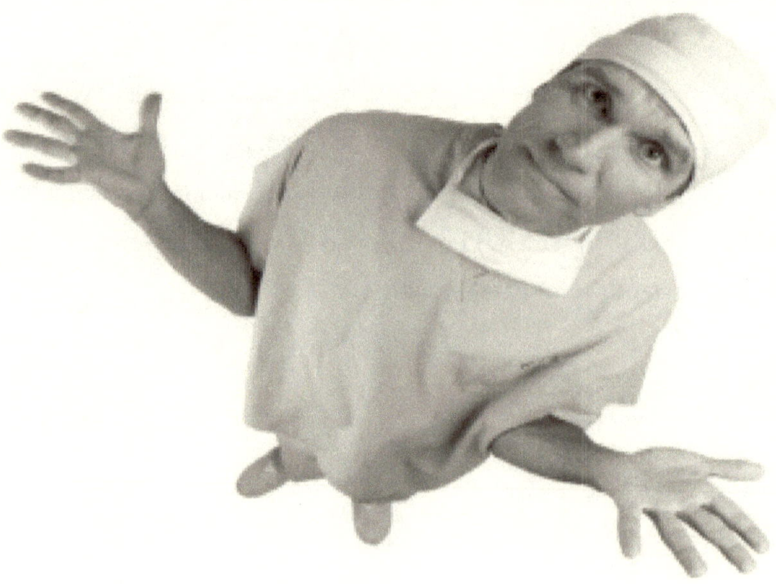

CBD Oil *might* help quell either of these chronic pains, since it has shown to have some action on the brain and nervous system. However, it's important to note that it does NOT help or treat the REASON WHY the pain exists, or help fix any structural or systemic problem. That's what pure nutritional supplements like Arthrosamine (for the joints), GI Support (for the digestive tract) can help with. More info on those can be found at MDsChoice.com

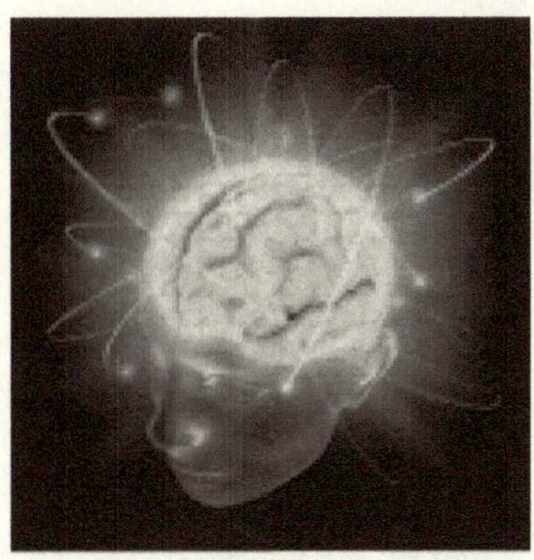

Some of the science surrounding CBD Oil and THC is seriously awesome, proving some elements are absolutely worth further study. Some of the advertising and marketing is claiming a mountain of capability based on a mole hill of actual facts.

Some of the claimed 'facts' are a complete illusion, marketed with the zeal of the old traveling snake oil salesman, selling a foul tasting alcohol laced herbal miracle cure, or remedy-everything potion, that *might* only temporarily mask the symptoms (usually dulled the senses, calmed the nerves, or blocked the pain) for just long enough for them to get out of town. They never really solved anything, except getting the money of unsuspecting people blind with hope, and often on the back of suffering, on false claims. Often perpetuating some common rumors, such as THC is natural to the body. It is not; cannabinoid is, which is absolutely different than THC.

These days, you find CBD Oils in products you can smoke, spray, eat, rub, drink, or even use sublingually (drops under the tongue), or even 'use' rectally.

**The problem is they are NOT all the same;
and really don't 'work' the same.**

Even from batch to batch from the same manufacturer, unless things are exactly the same... the concentration, potency, capability, and strength could easily be different from harvest to harvest, and batch to batch.

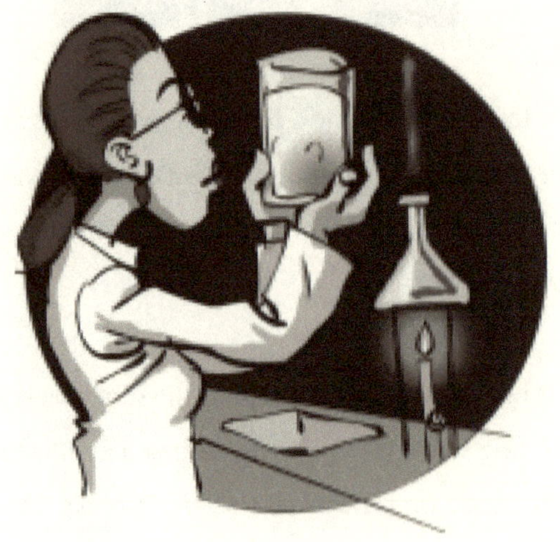

Page Intentionally Left Blank for Your Own Notes:

IS IT LEGAL?

"You have to know your local law." Is NOT the simple answer, or correct answer; because **there are many other factors to consider, such as federal laws, and the different INSURANCE RULES!** Which includes Workers Comp, life, auto, disability, and any that cover potential liability if there is an accident you might be party to someday. Remember, alcohol is legal, within certain boundaries, limits, and exceptions. And many of those laws vary state to state.

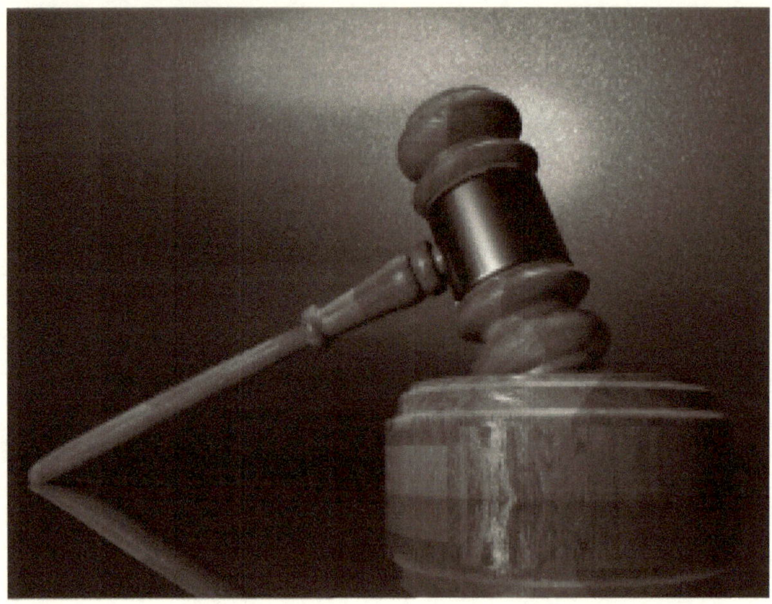

• **President Trump's "Right to Try"** Legislation, amends Federal law, to allow CERTAIN unapproved, experimental drugs to be administered to TERMINALLY ILL patients who have EXHAUSED ALL approved treatment options and unable to participate in clinical drug trials.

So many applauded President Trump's "Right To Try" Legislation, and while it was a step in the right direction that should have happened decades ago; honestly, it doesn't go far enough. It's ultimately like a pretty little sports car with a tiny two cylinder motor, 'all show, and no go.'

Currently, the Executive Order merely amends the Federal law to allow **certain** unapproved, experimental drugs to be administered to terminally ill patients who have exhausted all approved treatment options and are unable to participate in clinical drug trials. But there are some additional, very specific limitations, which totally eliminates all regular people with 'just chronic issues' that aren't immediately life threatening AND considered untreatable by, or unresponsive to, conventional medicine. It also matters whether or not they are officially being treated by a real doctor, who actually specializes in the field of study that relates to their particular terminal disease or diagnosis, is another factor.

So, while it 'sounds' good… and is a first (baby) step, it's pretty empty, and honestly impacts very few people in this nation.

Some other limits are:
- Eligible drugs **must have undergone** the Food and Drug Administration's (FDA) Phase I (safety) testing.
- The bill **requires any manufacturer or sponsor** of an eligible investigational drug to report to the FDA on any use of the drug on a "Right to Try" basis.

- FDA will post an annual summary report of "Right to Try" use on its website.
- The bill limits the liability of drug sponsors, manufacturers, prescribers, or dispensers that provide **or decline to provide** an eligible investigational drug to an eligible patient.

Whenever there is room for 'interpretation' in any government ruling, regulation, or law... there is room for argument, and two sides, with massive expenses and hassles!

• **Carly's Law** only applies to individuals with a debilitating illness who are enrolled in a FDA approved study by the University of Alabama-Birmingham, and the oil can only contain 3% tetrahydrocannabinol (THC).

• **Leni's Law** applies to only to people with debilitating illness that is specifically diagnosed by a doctor. The CBD oil can only contain up to 3 percent THC.

Drug enforcement is difficult without local state support. So, when a state legalizes recreational cannabis, and local law enforcement almost completely stops enforcing the prohibition, except for extreme situations, the Feds usually go along with what the locals decide. The states that have only 'medical use' legal, still enforce the laws against their citizens caught growing, selling, distributing, and using for recreational use – as it suits them.

However, law enforcement is not the only concern, or reality, even if it was legal in all 50 states.

Among the prohibitions are banking laws, and regulations, which specifically state that it is illegal (for the bank) to "knowingly engag[ing] in a monetary transaction in criminally derived property of value greater than $10,000." Most banks find it easier just to say "No thank you" than to gamble with feds enforcing any laws, particularly when they are FDIC insured; because being caught doing business with anyone the feds claim is a 'criminal enterprise' or 'obtained the money through any crime' could not only cost the bank huge fines, but their future.

It's 'legal' in Oregon, but they limit the number of plants, and randomly inspect the growing area of resellers for compliance (inspected for quantity, not quality). HOWEVER, when it comes to workplace drug testing, Oregon has a higher percentage of workplace drug tests that are positive for marijuana than any other state in the country. Employer can legally test employees for all drugs, including cannabis use, and FIRE THEM (or decline to hire them) if they test positive. More firms are reporting trouble finding workers who can pass a drug test.

Prior to December 20th, 2018's Farm Bill being passed and signed into law, in Alabama, CBD Oil was absolutely ILLEGAL – both federally, and under the state laws. On August 24th, 2018, just a few months ago, Chief Assistant Lauderdale County DA Angie Hamilton said, "It's time to put an end to the misconceptions about CBD Oil." She continued with, "CBD oil is unlawful. It is illegal for someone to possess it or distribute it," Hamilton said. For that reason, area officials announced a "crackdown" on CBD oil is underway in the region." Interestingly, Alabama State's government is listed as an official participant in the USDA hemp research pilot program, which allows them to choose who can grow and what happens with the product created in their state. The Farm Bill, at least until or unless it is changed again in the future, allows all Industrial Hemp, and products derived from JUST industrial hemp, to no longer be against Federal Law. That does NOT mean it might not still be against STATE LAWS, and penalties.

In Massachusetts, where you can now grow marijuana at home, it is still a crime to grow even hemp without a state license.

So, those boldly telling you 'It IS LEGAL in all 50 States' aren't going to be 'doing YOUR TIME, or paying YOUR FINES (or attorney costs), if you have a legal issue arising from any 'cannabis' product – made of marijuana or with too high of THC level.

Supposedly the NIK test, most often used in the field for most drugs isn't very accurate with any of the CBD Products. The federal government has backed off enforcing laws against marijuana and derivatives, including CBD, a great deal since January 21st, 2017 when President Trump took office, and the war became focused on disaster recovery, more vetting of immigrants, border control, the racial divide, defense security, and thanks to the media, we can't easily ignore President Trump's tweets. (Which often are a joke, purposefully inciting, intended to distract and be fodder to feed the media and his haters… with the skill of a master magician, as he presses through something else on the sidelines while they are all distracted by his often comical tweets).

Since the beginning of "The War on Drugs," the number of Americans incarcerated for drug offenses has soared from about 40,000 total in the entire nation, to well over ONE MILLION (county, state, and federally) for non-violent offenses, and the majority have no other criminal record. Acquittals become increasingly difficult to obtain, unless you have a pile of money and a great attorney experienced in dealing with drug cases. Today, the federal court system boasts over a 90% conviction rate. What are your odds? IF…

According to Anjelica Cappellino, J.D. in the Federal Courts in New York, "A study conducted by the Marijuana Policy Project demonstrated how over-the-counter Tylenol PM tested positive for cocaine, while Hershey's chocolate tested positive for marijuana. A host of other common household items can yield a positive result; for example, Mucinex may test positive for heroin and morphine, and soap can produce a false positive for GHB. "

Lawsuits against the drug testing manufacturer elicited this response, from the Safariland Group, which makes the NIK field tests (Narcotics Identification Kit) have stated, "These training materials, which outline protocols for use, clearly state that the tests are presumptive aids that serve only as confirmation of probable cause and are not a substitute for laboratory testing," the company wrote in a statement.

The New York Times found that tens of thousands of people are sent to jail each year based on the kits' results, which often generate false positives, for a variety of reasons. "Some tests ... use a single tube of a chemical called cobalt thiocyanate, which turns blue when it is exposed to cocaine. But cobalt thiocyanate also turns blue when it is exposed to more than 80 other compounds, including methadone, certain acne medications and several common household cleaners. Other tests use three tubes, which the officer can break in a specific order to rule out everything but the drug in question — but if the officer breaks the tubes in the wrong order, that, too, can invalidate the results. The environment can also present problems. Cold weather slows the color development; heat speeds it up, or sometimes prevents a color reaction from taking place at all."

The field tests for controlled substances aren't perfect. Like Luminol, used in serology, to test for the 'presents of blood' at suspected crime scenes, it doesn't determine who's blood it is, or if it is even really human blood. Apparently it also is known to give some false positives, with things like horseradish & copper.

If you are poor, and without quality legal representation, the system is often not fair, or always accurate. In the world of Hemp, cannabis, marijuana, and all the products derived from those plants, there is a growing collision, association, and group that is pushing for scientific studies, legalization, and decriminalization. One such group is the HIA (Hemp Industry Association), which have filed a key law suits on behalf of 'the industry.' Interestingly, the judges that shot down the HIA's appeal acknowledged the Farm bill's definition of 'legal cannabis' absolutely differs from the DEA's. The judge further acknowledged the conflict between the CSA (Controlled Substance Act) and FB (Farm Bill).

"We're in this stage where we have non-enforcement at the federal level, non-enforcement at the state level," says Cristina Buccola, a New York-based attorney who advises cannabis-related businesses. "For all intents and purposes it looks like a legal substance." [But it technically, and federally, IS NOT... yet]

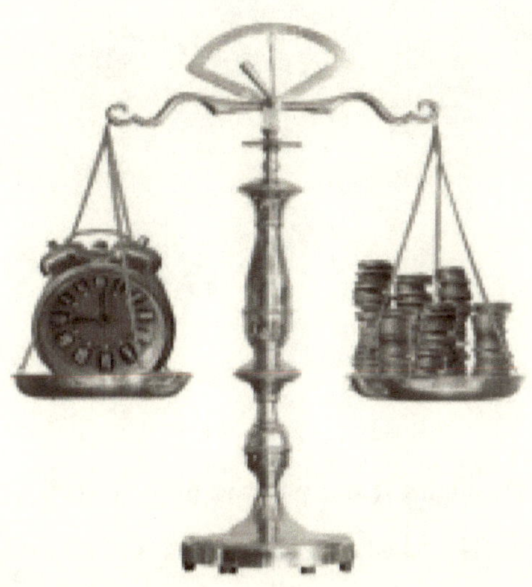

HIA vs DEA, 2001, published a rule regarding industrial hemp products in the Federal Register, banning hemp seed and oil food products that contain ANY amount of THC.

The HIA (Hemp Industries Association) sued in the 9ᵗʰ Circuit Court of Appeals, to get a stay. According to the official Health CANADA Testing protocol, the hemp food companies' products generally did not have any detectable THC, they argued. [Remember, all hemp products have SOME, albeit fractional < 0.3% supposedly]. The argument about the testing, is they are in the United States... trying to apply a Canadian testing protocol.

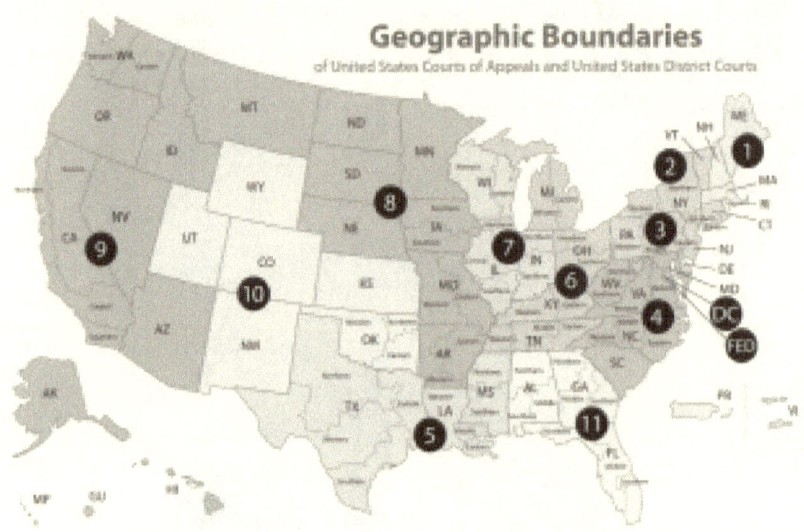

Which basically means that if you live in the jurisdiction of the 9th Circuit Court of Appeals (Alaska, Washington, Oregon, California, Arizona, Idaho, Montana, Nevada, Guam, Northern Mariana Islands), and have an issue with marijuana, or virtually any cannabis product, especially in one of those 'legal states,' you are less likely to have federal intervention or anything more than a ticket and fine, unless they believe you are part of a criminal enterprise, gang activity, harming children, or killing adults.

In the other districts, attorneys are attempting to use the 9th Circuit Court of Appeals ruling as precedent, with varying success. Until, and unless, it goes to the SCOTUS (Supreme Court of the United States), it will remain a variable for each state, and then each district in the state, assuming a 'guilty' verdict is appeal or a writ is filed to get relief through the courts.

In 2003, the DEA revised their ban, to '**any amount of trace residual THC.**' Since all hemp derived from cannabis has at least a fractional amount, they officially banned ALL HEMP from being imported for processing and manufacturing in the USA. That destroyed many American companies, both those growing industrial hemp, and those making a variety of products from body care to nutritional products. So, another law suit.

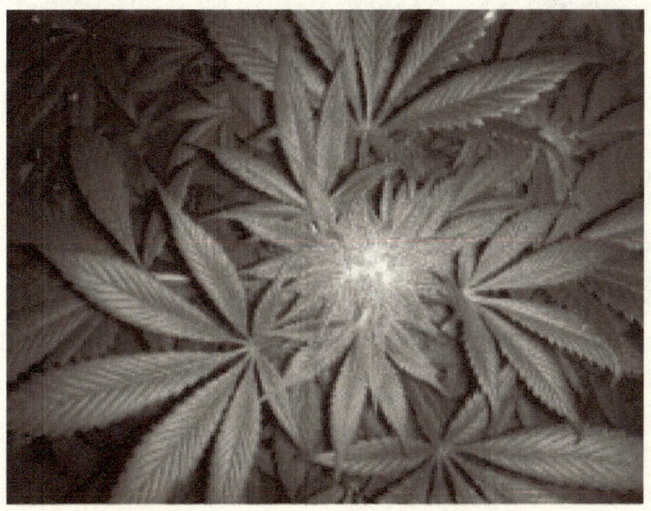

On May 22nd, 2018, the DEA (Drug Enforcement Agency) released an internal directive that makes a key point: "Products and materials that are made from the cannabis plant and **which fall outside the CSA definition of marijuana** are not controlled under the CSA. Such products may accordingly be sold and otherwise distributed throughout the United States without restriction under the CSA or its implementing regulations. The mere presence of cannabinoids is not itself dispositive as to whether a substance is within the scope of the CSA;"

This time with the 9th Circuit issuing a unanimous decision in favor of the HIA, where Judge Betty Fletcher wrote, "[T]hey (DEA) cannot regulate naturally occurring THC not contained within or derived from marijuana – i.e. non-psychoactive hemp is not included in Schedule 1. The DEA has no authority to regulate drugs that are not scheduled, and it has not followed procedure required to schedule a substance. The DEA's definition of "THC" contravenes the unambiguously expressed intent of Congress in the Controlled Substances Act (SCA) and cannot be upheld". September 28th, 2004, the HIA claimed victory, after the DEA declined to appeal to the SCOTUS (Supreme Court of the United States).

However, that was 2004. Understand, right now today, fourteen years after that decision, Industrial hemp remains legal for import and sale in the USA, but America farmers are still not permitted to grow it without special DEA, FDA, and USDA waivers, exemptions, and approval. So, that 'interpretation' has some clear lines, that remain gray... and is ultimately tied to both THC levels found, using whatever test they choose to use, AND the amount of time, resources, and money one (or a group) has to fight.

The results of the Ninth Circuit Court of Appeals ruling stands still today. Enjoining (slowing to stopping) the FEDERAL DOJ from enforcement of what is now 21 C.F.R. § 1308.11(d)(31) (drug code 7370) with respect to products that are excluded from the definition of marijuana in the Controlled Substances Act (CSA). The inferred meaning is that if it isn't specifically and directly mentioned, listed, or with cause... it's to be 'left alone' by the DOJ (Department of Justice).

Today, because of that ruling, the DEA generally does not enforce that provision of the law, regarding such products. Note: it says: DOES NOT ENFORCE, not 'It is Legal' – and only limits the DOJ (federal justice system), and has zero impact on the state systems - which is significant and key, if there ever were legal questions or concerns.

Also, notice that it does NOT name or list any specific products they 'aren't enforcing the laws on,' which leaves a huge gray area when you consider 'which fall outside the CSA definition of marijuana.' More legalese, and another ambiguous phrase subject to legal interpretation, in court, should any law enforcement agency want to make an issue of something. The fight is not over, and little is really settled.

So the answer to the question, "Is it legal?" Is NO, according to the DEA, FDA, and even most in the USDA! Even if it's deemed 'legal' in your state.

If something happened and you were 'caught' with it on federal property, the post office or a national park, or a state that hasn't implicitly legalized it, you would be breaking the law, and subject to arrest if that officer so decided to enforce that law. **Be aware of just what the rules are regarding use, possession, and distribution.**

YES! PEOPLE HAVE BEEN ARRESTED in 2018 for 'possession' and 'possession with intent' [to distribute] for JUST CBD OIL! Those that could afford attorneys are reportedly 'beating' the charges, or able to get them significantly reduced, sometimes even dropped, like Mamadou Ndiaye in Indiana. However, people like Anita Maddux, jailed in Jackson Hole, Wyoming, is still pending resolution. The Teton County jail personnel found her CBD oil and used a NIK test to determine the presence of THC. She was arrested, told she could leave if she 'promised to appear' AND pay an $850 bond. She was from out of state, and didn't have the money, so in jail she's remained in jail pending a court decision.

On August 3rd (2018) a man in Cary Indiana, for 241 pounds of CBD Gummies... arrested. His case is still in process, as of today (the initial release of this book).

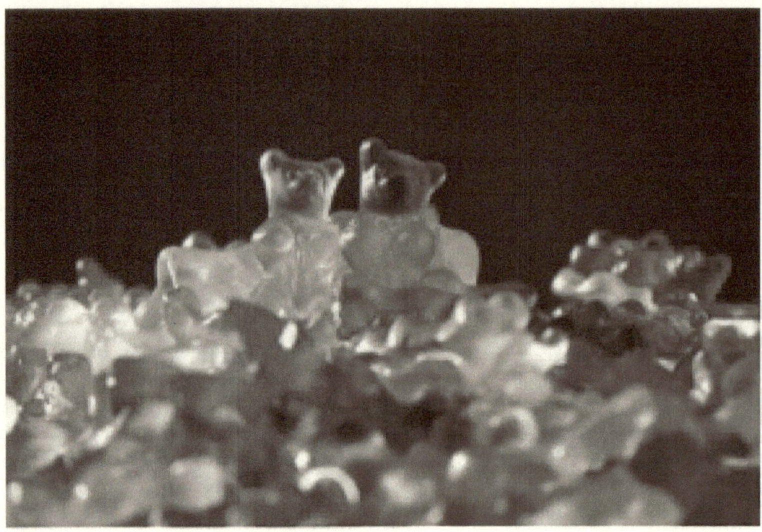

The Rohrabacher-Farr amendment must be renewed every year, for states to generally have some 'say' as to the legality of marijuana (and cannabis derived products) within their state borders. Until I started researching for this book, I didn't realize this. That renewal has, thus far, happened each year, since 2010.

October 2018, Alan Gordon, 48, and Anne Armstrong, 58, - who are running for Rhode Island attorney general and governor, respectively - were arrested for having 48 pounds of marijuana. They were running on the 'Compassion Party' ticket, and are leaders of some religious group, 'The Healing Church' that uses marijuana for religious services. Since their 15yr old child was in the house, the state took their child and filed 'contributing to the delinquency of a minor' charges, in addition to 'possession' charges.

However, understand, if it is ever not renewed, or otherwise allowed to expire, then all state protections vanish; and the DEA, FDA, USDA, FBI, and DHLS could have free reign to bust anyone for possession, sale, growing, use, or whatever. Right now, today, it is mostly up to the states, unless you are deemed part of a gang, possessing with the intent to sell, or otherwise manufacturing without authorization or necessary approval, it is technically and really illegal on the federal level.

Only the 'for recreational use' states have pretty much ceased arrests and prosecution for cannabis related crimes. It is important to understand that Rohrabacher-Blumenauer only **prohibits the DOJ from using federal funds to interfere with state-legal marijuana laws** and companies.

It does NOT prevent them from 'acting upon law breakers.' It merely creates a speed bump, of various sizes (depending on the state), blocking the Feds from 'using federal funds to INTERFERE' (so, the state can request their assistance, and interstate commerce can supersede the limits, along with a few other technicalities).

Don't forget those states, counties, and agencies that love 'civil forfiture.' (If you don't know what it is, look it up... the reality of unconstitutionally should help enlighten you, as there is no Due Process, or civil rights protections for most citizens.) So, do not count your chickens, yet.

Even in 'legal' states, the rules are varied, and are subject to change at the whim of politicians. Technically, you cannot legally give it to anyone outside your household, except in the 'recreational states' and then subject to the states limits.

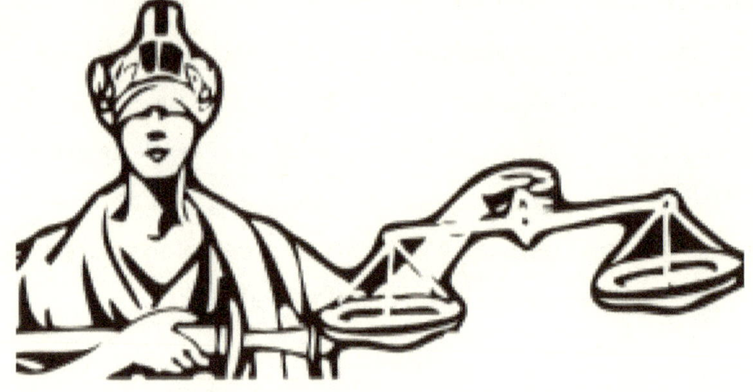

In 2016, Chuck Rosenberg, Acting Administrator of the DOJ (Department of Justice), DEA (Drug Enforcement Administration), wrote a relatively famous letter to a couple judges (Rhode Island and Washington States) and another individual (Bryan Krumm, redacted location). Key points to that official letter:

1) **DOJ, DEA, FDA, and USDA all work together [in the 'War on Drugs'],** and control all official 'research' on marijuana and CBD in the United States, and have been for years. They currently have approved 354 'individuals and institutions' with their registration

process, to grow and research [note: there is NO MENTION of 'SELL' or 'distribute' in their memo]…

2) Acknowledgement of WAIVER for certain regulatory requirements for approved researchers conducting **FDA authorized trials on cannabidiol (CBD).** [which means they absolutely and clearly believe that CBD falls under their CSA Schedule 1 mandate].

3) CBD studies 'have shown promise' for the treatment of a specific medical condition, such as childhood epilepsy. [Again, reminding people THEY have the control over the CBD industry, as well as cannabis at large; and expect 'safety' studies, and 'functional use' studies, to justify medical use]. And,

4) "We believe that the drug approval process is the proper way to assess whether a product derived from marijuana or its constituent parts is safe and effective for medical use." seals the deal. They are demanding official, documented, peer reviewed testing, studies, and are indirectly promoting Big Pharma, which are the only groups that can afford to play that game, in the name of 'public safety.' [**FYI: it's estimated that the average FDA 'drug approval' costs nearly $1 Billion dollars, and generally takes 2 to 7 years to *maybe* get approval,** unless you're part of big pharma. Even then, their 'approval' does not prove 'it works'… or works as intended, or does not have dangerous side effects, but rather that it 'appears safe under certain conditions.']

Today, with the DEA choosing NOT TO ENFORCE a law does NOT mean that it is legal, that the law has actually changed because some states legalized things, to some level, or that it is not subject to change (one way or the other) at a moment's notice. When the FDA approves a drug (for use), and establishes how it can be used, they also limit what CAN BE said about a given product, and mandates certain things that MUST BE said. Then the DEA creates regulatory tracking number, any necessary exemptions for that drug, and 'used within' parameters.

Hemp Farming Act of 2018 - S.2667 - 115th Congress (2017-2018) – handily passed in the Senate 86-11 on June 28, 2018 to get a door open for legalizing farmers and growers of INDUSTRIAL hemp in the USA without special approval, or the hassles of endless paperwork most have to go through today. Sponsored by Sen Mitch McConnell, R-Kentucky, where a legal research grow has been happening in the shadows of the University for a few years now.

The passing of that bill does not 'legalize' pot, it is just another step in that direction, and a sign of the absolute softening of opinion on the topic, by both the citizens of this nation and the government officials (even the staunch GOP conservatives).

October 17th, 2018, ALL MARIJUANA became 100% legal in the entire country of Canada! Uruguay was the first country to completely legalize it, in 2017. After years of planning (cough, how the government could regulate and profit from it). The national 'recreational' legalization approach has nearly eliminated the black market, put a serious dent in crime, and allowed for national banking, just like any legal business. The all shipments of cannabis (and cannabis products) without restrictions, online ordering, postal delivery, billions of dollars in investment, and unrestricted scientific studies.

National prohibition in the U.S. is shifting, and it will be federally legal in our lifetime! For the same reasons as Canada & Uruguay. **It has been projected that cannabis products will be legal for medical use federally in the USA, and most of the 50 states, before 2024,** unless something drastic happens. The **December 20th 2018 Farm Bill was THE START… removing Industrial Hemp and CBD Oil** made from **such hemp from the Federal Controlled Substance Schedules,** and thus no longer officially and blatantly against Federal Law.

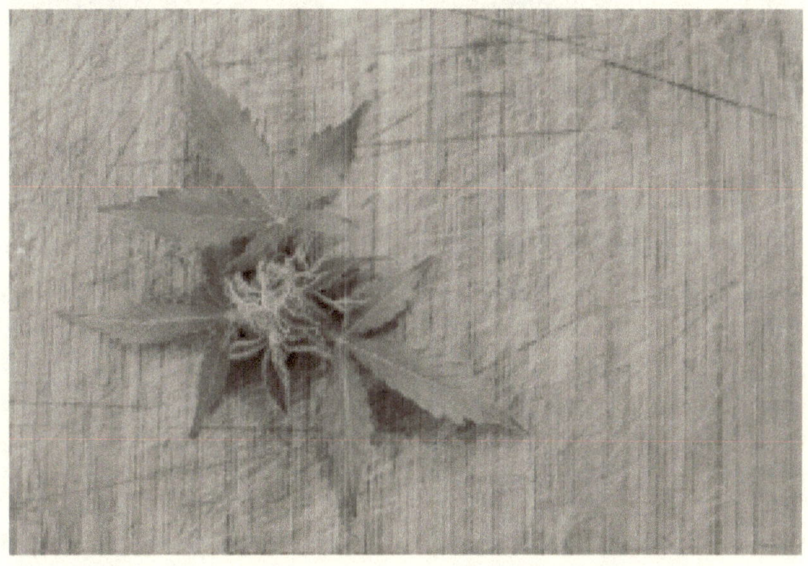

Pew Research Center, January 2018, said over 61% of the surveyed American Citizens 'think weed should be legalized.' Gallup Polls say over 64% of the American Citizens are now in favor of legalization, and over 51% for Republicans for the first time ever! Note that both those polls show a higher approval rating than even 1969 when the tracking of opinions on marijuana officially started.

So, more states will be pushing to legalize medical and personal recreational use, because citizens are tired of being told 'no,' 'they can't,' and don't want to see family and friends punished for using cannabis (especially those with chronic or serious medical reasons which a cannabis type product might help treat).

Projections show that the federal government will officially, and finally, remove marijuana (and all other cannabis products) from the Schedule 1 list before the end of 2025. That will be huge; and will absolutely impact the alcohol market, and big pharma... which have likely been busy lobbying against such legalization for the last few decades. Legalization will impact virtually every citizen in this nation, especially those that suffer from something it *might* help (or just wants an alternative to alcohol or prescription pain killers). Decriminalization is NOT the same as 'legalization' ... and it will not alter how the FDA deals with claims.

If you are in a state that it is 'legal' – then odds are, at the state level, it will be treated much like alcohol already is, as the state collects taxes, permit fees, and fines for those over stepping their laws and rules. **If you do not have intoxicating levels in your system at the time of the incident, and were not indulging at the time, it is not likely to be a problem the legal states.**

In Colorado alone, cannabis product related sales reached $996m in just 2015, and raked in $135m in tax revenue. In 2017, those numbers were $1.5b in sales, and upwards of $247 million in taxes and fees collected by the government. (That is **OVER $5 Billion in tax revenue on the legal sales, in just Colorado, in the first four years it was legalized**).

They use the money for road improvements, recreation centers for both children and adults, and scholarships for low-income students. Now, with that much money in play, investors and pro-cannabis special interest groups have begun to flex their political muscles; to help ensure things remain legal (at least in their state, to the best of their ability). Pro-pot lobbyists in Denver are now battling on some equal footing with their counterparts in the pharmaceutical, alcohol, judicial and prison industries that want to keep cannabis products criminalized.

Today, because it is 'derived from cannabis' it is absolutely against Federal law. So, I would be careful assuming you're 'golden' (or in the clear), unless you have a pile of money and a great attorney **IF anything ever come up**, or the wrong person in power wants to try to make an example out of you (or your use).

This is not some 'scare tactic,' it is reality. Like '11 over the speed limit,' most people will not be stopped, fined, or hassled by traffic cops… unless they are in a school zone, driving dangerously, or they were already involved in an accident.

However, every once in a while, laws often 'over looked' get enforced, fines and arrests are made for lesser offenses.

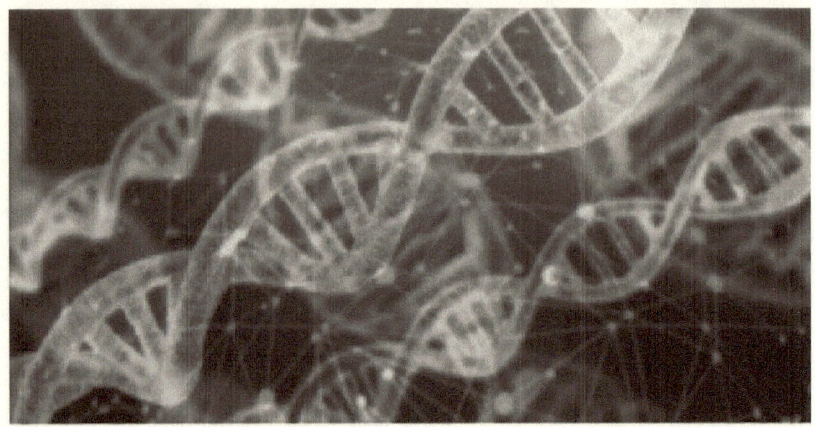

Remember, alcohol is legal (if you're over 21), but if you're intoxicated and your actions cause someone to be harmed or other people's property to be damaged… your guilt, punishment, and culpability will likely be higher… and the resources available to help you will likely be fewer. So, thinking 'it's legal' even if you are living in one of the states that have legalized recreational use, does not mean you cannot still have legal problems if you are intoxicated or testing positive for it 'in your system' if stuff goes sideways.

The fact is that some sales people and companies are claiming CBD's legality depends completely upon the THC content, but does it, really? **NOPE!** Especially not before November 2018's Farm Bill. Now, so long as it is derived from INDUSTRIAL HEMP and not making medical claims, it *might* be legal in most states. There are 33 states, with existing rules, that should allow some leniency and use, under their rules. Check with YOUR STATE officials, and GET IT IN WRITING!

Effective in January 2017, the DEA (which typically refers to marijuana by the plant's scientific species name, Cannabis sativa, or the Reefer Madness-era spelling "marihuana" or the more modern 'marijuana' spelling) **made an official ruling stating that "the marijuana scheduling includes 'marihuana extract.'" To be further specific, in the rule, the agency defined "marihuana extract" as** any "extract containing one or more cannabinoids _that has been derived from any plant of the genus Cannabis_"**—which absolutely includes CBD (the Farm Bill of 2018 removed 'Industrial Hemp' and products derived from that form of cannabis, from the Schedule 1 listings, but slapped all medical use directly under the FDA for regulations, and scientific requirements.**

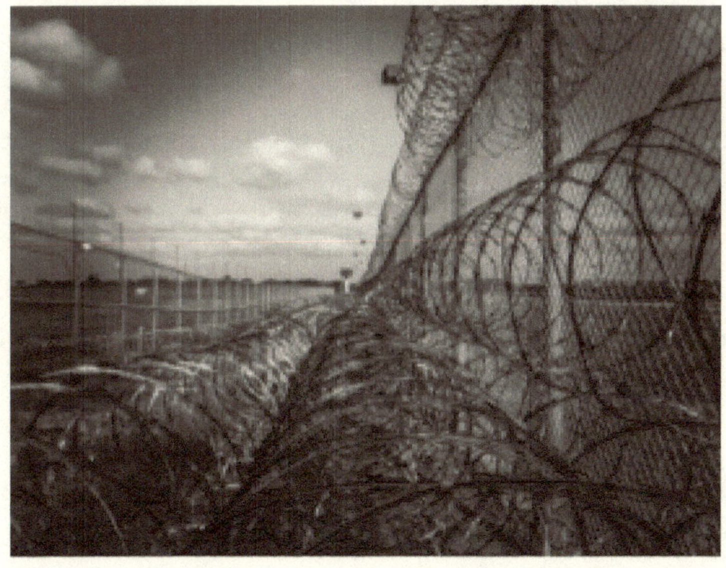

Those people saying it is 100% legal in all states, are 100% wrong! They are purposefully ignoring FEDERAL LAWS prior to November 2018… and are still subject to limitations, regulations, and STATE LAWS. And if there is more than 0.03% THC OR they are talking about any 'cures' (prevention or treatments) without absolute science on THEIR BRAND/FORM then they are ignoring all the laws the FDA has long established.

"CBD oil with less than .3% THC will not likely show up on a standard drug test, with normal dosing." That *might* be a true statement. HOWEVER, we have spoke with quite a few manufacturers that say there is ZERO PERCENT THC in 'the CBD Oil' they are selling, and when pushed for a LEGAL INDEMNIFICATION, they admitted they were lying!

When pushed, each admitted that there was either 'some' (less than 1% usually) which they claim 'wouldn't likely show up on a test.' OR that their product 'really' was NOT derived from cannabis, but some HERBAL CONCOCTION that (they claimed) reacted 'like' CBD or marijuana (huge difference, really and scientifically).

There is no such thing as absolutely 0% THC in CBD oil, it is physically impossible it if was really made from a cannabis based product. Just like there is no such thing as 100% pure Gold...

The really high-quality CBD is 0.3% THC content, or less, which is unlikely to show in a standard blood or urine test at normal dosing (if you take high doses, you could have more of a buildup in your system). Why the sales people can't be honest is mind boggling. Maybe they don't know. Maybe they just don't care, and are just out to make the quick buck, while they can.

However, there is a lot of inexpensively made product that has tested out at 3-5%, which is a huge difference, which can show (in most drug tests, depending on your dose and method of use). You have to ask, just how positive you are that there really is LOW THC, if a test is ever legally demanded. And, do you care? Does it matter to your life… your future?

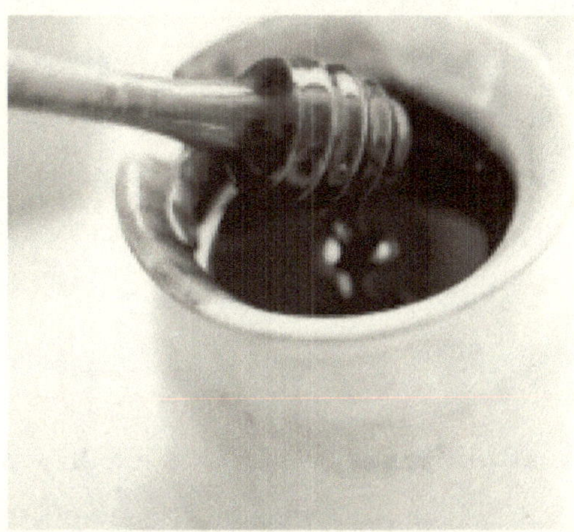

THC is a component of real CBD oil, which necessarily comes from cannabis. Think of it like a watermelon, even the seedless varieties have seeds – just not as many. The THC level is determined by the starting cannabis plant AND the processing. Those are the key factors that establish how much THC is really in the CBD oil. The quality and consistency of the manufacturing process is important, and ultimately impactful to the purpose, use, and goals.

We have seen CBD Oils being sold with claimed levels from 100mg per bottle, per ml (per eye dropper), per gel cap, per gummy, and supposedly even per drop. (The latter are generally much more expensive, but stronger 'per dose' is usually the purest, if it is accurate, and really at that level).

The likelihood you will be hassled over a cannabis product, including CBD, really depends on the state, and the situation.

CBD oil in Virginia is technically legal, so long as it contains less than 5% THC; however, just across the border in South Carolina, anything over 0.9% THC is illegal to possess. But remember, those are state laws, and the absolute reality (today) is that it is **ALL is still illegal according to the Federal Law at any THC level (even if absolute zero, if there was such a thing)**, merely because of the way the Schedule 1 listing is written. If it is a 'component of' a cannabis plant that is meant to be 'taken' (smoked, vaped, swallowed, or rubbed on), all things the FDA has oversight on at this time.

Any and all 'claims' of prevention, treatment, or cure have a slew of federal laws that must be complied with by the manufacturers and marketers; and the majority peddling product today are ignoring all that; which makes it even easier for the fake stuff to get mixed in. These are very real legal technicalities most CBD Oil manufacturers and sellers have not been hit hard with, yet. But rest assured, right or wrong, good or bad, they will be, eventually. The FDA is watching!

Even ibuprofen and vitamin C are both regulated by the FDA, and the claims used in marketing them have some absolute restrictions. There are a whole lot of people pushing CBD Oils, and Hemp Oils, that clearly don't know anything about the government laws and regulations, or they just don't care... or somehow think they are exempt, likely falsely believing 'the laws' don't apply to THEIR product.

CBD, once approved federally, will absolutely will be regulated by the DSHEA rules and the FDA. Like gold, there will be some 'industry standards' established, so people can understand what is actually in the product they are buying (something that doesn't honestly exist, really, today). The oversight is just a matter of time, delayed because it is still technically illegal at the federal level, under the CSA.

The problem is there is little consistency in manufacturing, especially between brands, but even harvest to harvest; they are not 'all the same.' They don't have any actual guidelines or regulations at this point, and some manufacturers (and sales people) employ little honesty, or scientific knowledge of what is 'in' their product. Some processed some type of hemp components into oil, using some method, but often seem to ignore other chemicals in 'the finished product.' Variables; from harvest to harvest, batch to batch, and company to company.

The vast majority of the products out there are 'cut' (diluted) with sweet almond oil, coconut oils, sesame seed oil, flaxseed oil, fish oil (omega 3 fatty acids), hemp oil, PG, VG, or some other 'food grade' consumable intended to dilute more expensive active ingredients. Among sales people pushing CBD Oil, **many are really unaware of all the actual ingredients used in the product they are selling**; or even how the oils are extracted. They do not really know what the laws actually are, or how their product may (or may not) really work in a body. **They are selling 'cures' (which might be completely untrue, and not really apply to their product).**

Many are using the valid science, that really proves something about 'CBD Oil' (and/or THC, and/or other cannabinoids) then CLAIMING that science applies to their product, and 'is the same' as what they are selling. That is often and usually not true. Until, or unless, the studies release more details about the EXACT FORMULA they used to achieve their results, and the study can be duplicated with a product from a different manufacturer, or the exact same Certificate of Analysis ingredients, expect a difference, from subtle to massive.

However, just like the TV promoter, Dr. Barefoot, did with 'Coral Calcium' a few years ago, before the FTC (Federal Trade Commission) stepped in with the FDA, to shut him down with some massive fines, he was making true statements about the science about what certain types of calcium, in certain studies, but were absolutely false claims about the type (form) of calcium HE WAS SELLING (and it really wasn't even 'coral' which is illegal to harvest).

Sort of like describing the transportation and delivery capability of a semi-truck, but delivering a 'smart car' or bicycle, or even just wheels without bearings... in place of what was described. It is marketing magic, in a world where the buyer must beware, or they will be scammed.

We have seen test results (COA) of a few different brands of CBD... with very different results, despite 'the same' label and marketing claims. That should be a concern to most end users and buyers, but it is usually 'after the fact.'

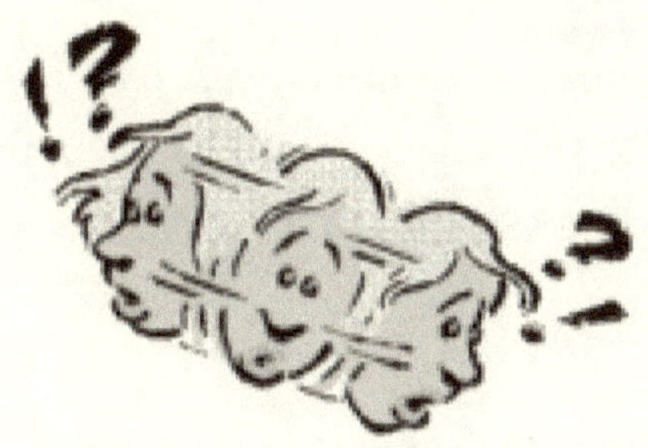

Just a call from a 'manufacturer' September 2018, wanting us to 'pick up' his product to add to our line of products we sell to resellers. He claimed to have three manufacturing facilities and distribution outlets in three different states. With his broken English foreign accent, he was trying to sell CBD Oil, for us to re-distribute to our customers. I told him I was actually editing a book I have been writing ON THE TOPIC, and was interested in hearing what he had to offer.

His next statement was interesting, and changed the entire tone of the conversation, when he claimed the CBD oil he was manufacturing was 0% THC, and 100% legal in all 50 states. (mind you, this happened multiple times in 2017 and 2018, prior to October 17th, 2018... before the Farm Bill was signed into law).

I asked to see the COA (Certificate Of Analysis), which he emailed. I noticed there was no line (or test results listed) for THC. So, I asked why,

He said, "There is Zero, so we don't test for it."

I asked what it was made out of, and he told me 'Industrial Hemp, with zero THC.'
When I reminded him I was actually working on a book on the topic, as

we speak (the manuscript was literally open on my computer at the time), and that **ALL HEMP contains THC. I told him, that if that wasn't a true statement, PLEASE PROVE IT… so I can be absolutely correct in my book.**

He started back peddling, then claiming that it was actually just 0.3%. 'and wouldn't test positive for THC, so they leave it off' (claiming ZERO on the label)

Although, using a normal dose *probably* will not show up in a blood test, the math matters. Consider, if they were edibles, who only eats just one? Or doses perfectly every time?

When I asked why the COA did not show THAT (level of THC). He started tap dancing around the truth again.

Next, when I asked him about potency, he told me they had 100mg and 1000mg strength doses to choose from. (I was doubtful; particularly at the prices he sent over)

So, I asked directly, if milligram listing was per bottle or milliliter. He admitted it was per bottle. (The problem with 100mg per bottle is that is only 3.333mg per ml (per eye dropper), at best. A far cry from the 100mg the label and the salesman were stating. The 1000mg per bottle is only 33.33mg per ml.

Understand the level needed for the average person, and those trying to treat a disease or issue are significantly different. The doses used in most studies to actually 'treat' something is usually 100mg to 600mg PER DAY! Not 'per month' or per bottle. And usually with some ratio of THC and OTHER cannabinoids included also – 'the full spectrum' of the plant.)

He repeated that his CBD Oil was legal in all 50 states (which was 100% untrue at that time).

When I asked him if he could produce a form in writing stating that, and would give me a Letter of Indemnification, and an Insurance Rider covering MY business from any legal action, claims or liability if we picked up that product to use or resell… he started hymning and hawing around.

I asked him if his company had federal approval, he said yes (without pause).

When I asked for proof, he said he'd have to talk with the owner of the company.

I asked how they got around the current Schedule 1 federal listing, banning 'all cannabis products' **HE HUNG UP ON ME!** (He knew it was REALLY ILLEGAL, and currently just 'unenforced' in most states, if the THC levels are 0.3% or less)

Wrap your head around that conversation. I have had a few discussions and conversations just like that one, over the last couple years.

With other manufacturers, other sales representatives. **Often, it is just a matter of knowing what questions to ask, and knowing some of the absolute truths to assertively determine if the sales-person is lying, telling the truth, or just ignorant.** Only a couple that I have had the opportunity to speak with have seemed to be 99.9% straight up, honest, and real… with some actual science, and a full spectrum COA on their product (which they were proud of, as they should have been).

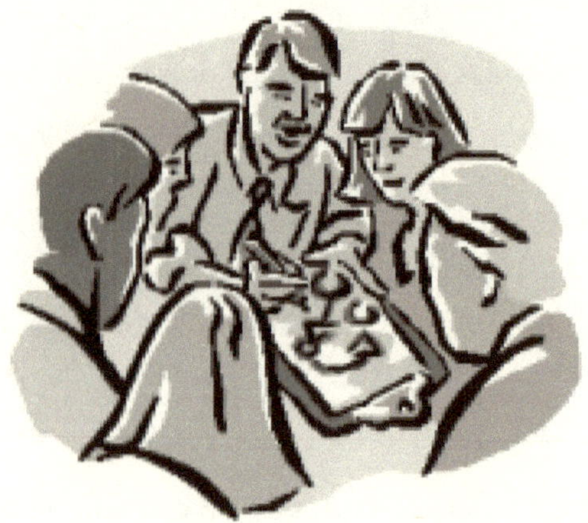

There is no such thing as 0% THC in a CBD Oil product made from cannabis, it is part of the DNA. Even the great stuff should have at least a fraction of a percent, .01 to .3%, but never 0%, not really.

So ANY sales person telling you a cannabis product has 0%, are either lying, or ignorant, or both! Or it is source is not really from the 'cannabis' family of plants. Period.

I have found no science or proof to the contrary of that statement, nor has any COA I've seen proven otherwise; I've asked, and searched.

However, with CBD Oil, the differences in medical application can be immense. Many of the studies, particularly on cancer, include a ratio level of THC, but I have noticed that none of the CBD manufacturers calling us – here in Tennessee - are mentioning that fact.

Knowing the actual ingredients, and the source of the CBD is vital, as well as the other stuff added, and what was used to dilute it. The cheap stuff can include other impurities, usually has less testing, and/or fewer safety measures.

The fundamental problem is that there are more levels, more variables, and most of the ingredients end up in the blood stream, brain, and spinal system… and might well create some other reactions, or side effects, depending on what they really are (and aren't).

Conclusion: Today, it is absolutely against federal law, and even in legal states have some valid concerns. IF you decide to use it anyway, then KNOW THE PURITY and POTENCY of the stuff you are using. Your life, life of your loved one, the health, and longevity could depend on it.

Today, there are only FOUR cannabis-based medical and health related products currently approved by the FDA and dispensed through a prescription. ALL others 'making claims' are technically (and absolutely) against Federal Law, under CSA Schedule 1, regardless of the state law.

No exceptions, only unenforced existing laws, with most officials willing to look the other direction, most of the time, especially if the state is profiting through the collection of taxes, permits, and other fees. The citizens of that state voted to legalize it, either for medical use or recreationally, but have not pushed the right buttons to get Federal approval, or FDA oversight. It will happen, probably soon.

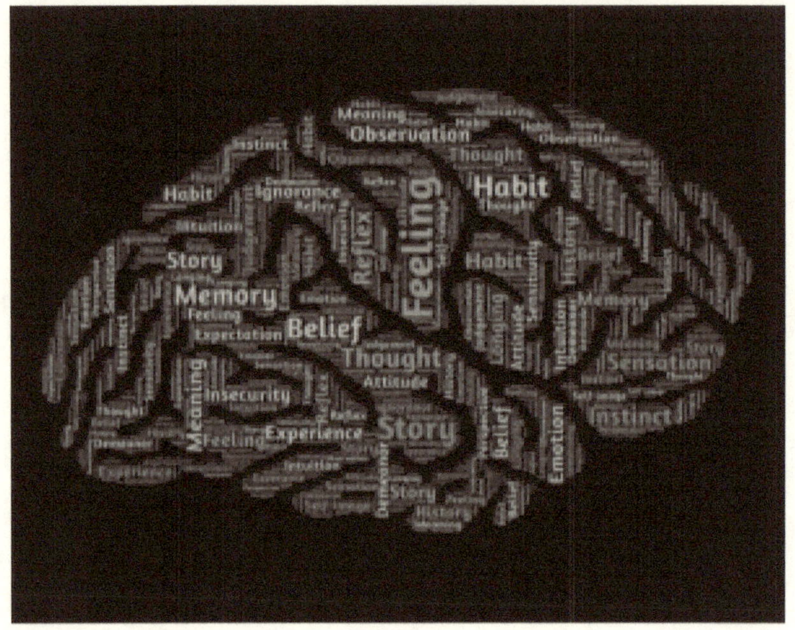

The DEA and FDA still, technically, have legal jurisdiction, if they choose to enforce it... even in the legal states. Though they there is little record of them pushing much since 2017, unless they suspect gang or organized crime activity. There have been a few raids of 'grows' and even swap meets, flea markets, and stores carrying CBD Oil, especially synthetics, in 2018. **But it does still happen.**

They are currently less likely to push things in the legal states, and more states are will create some type of pro-cannabis legislation in 2020 and 2024. As the citizen's approval (or passive acceptance) continues to rise.

There will be 'some' THC in all CBD Oils made from cannabis plants. The question is HOW MUCH, REALLY: Then, the math to figure out how many milligrams there actually are per milliliters, and what it's cut with... and if there are any other additives, or impurities. It is important to know if they are actually testing it from batch to batch (because the results will vary, and some will absolutely be there!). Their COA (Certificate of Analysis) is very important, and not often shared, or public information. If you do get to see a real COA, it should include the date, batch number, all components tested for, and the results... in mg, ng, ml, ppm (parts per million), or ppb (parts per billion) of each component.

Today, Canada has deemed 10ppm THC as a 'safe limit' in their testing. In general, Hemp oil contains less than 25ppm CBD, while the marijuana based extracted CBD will be significantly higher than those numbers, and ultimately depends on the strain and part of the plant used to harvest it. Also, **check to see IF THC is even actually tested for (the lack of that line item, on tests, or a claim of absolute 0% or 0ppb (parts per billion) should both be quite telling.**

At this time, the manufacturer has little liability for any 'mistake' or omission in actual THC levels, or toxins (like heavy metals), found in their product, because there are absolutely no regulations... no protocols, other than some resellers claiming it's a 'dietary supplement' that falls under DSHEA (Dietary Supplement Health and Education Act of 1994).

If push comes to shove, most will claim anything negative found in your blood or urine is YOUR FAULT (claiming it 'didn't come from their product). Especially if you have any legal issue, or lose any insurance claim, benefits, or are somehow found to have too much THC in your system in any type of legal dispute.

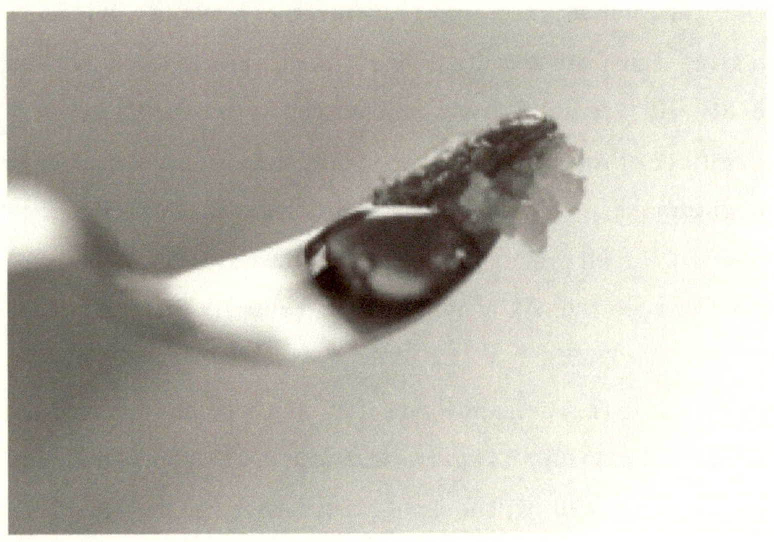

The problem is the cost of the testing… and WHEN it is tested (you want on finished product… not raw materials!)

Proving the COA came from THEIR PRODUCT, and is done on each LOT (batch) could be expensive, time consuming, but is vital to effective safety.

If there is a legal problem, it is likely and ultimately like getting blood out of that proverbial turnip, with most manufacturer's protected by layers of denial, unless they are a big or well established business that is doing the extraction, testing, mixing, and testing on the finished product.

Regardless of WHERE you bought it, the majority of the companies making CBD Oils today are relatively small businesses, and couldn't weather any large civil lawsuits if they screwed up.

Ultimately, it is Buyer Beware.

If you are thinking of growing, investing, or otherwise getting involved with or in cannabis, marijuana, or CBD products… you need to pay particularly close attention to 'How It All Started' section)

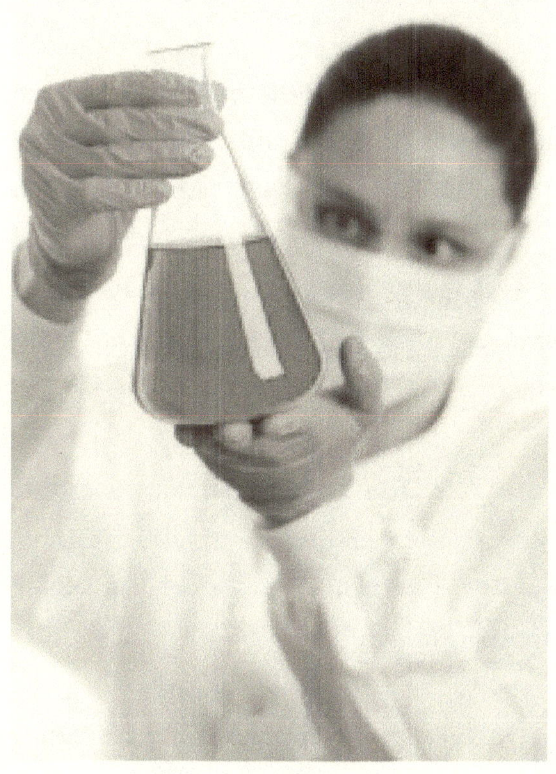

BIGGEST CONCERN:

As of the November 2018 elections, twenty three states and DC have legalized medical marijuana, and 10 states (Alaska, California, Colorado, Maine, Massachusetts, Michigan, Nevada, Oregon, Vermont, and Washington) plus the District of Columbia and Northern Mariana Islands have legalized recreational use. Fourteen of the states, plus the US Virgin Islands, has completely decriminalized it. **That's a total of 33 states that claim it is 'ok' – or at least not an issue from the state.**

According to the DEA, FDA, FBI, and federal government, 'cannabis sativa' is still illegal in all 50 states and territories at the federal level; only Industrial-Hemp, after December 20th, 2018 has been removed from the FEDERAL Controlled Substance Schedules, but still subject to STATE LAWS (as there are no Constitutional Protections). This reality has created a great deal of tension between the state and federal levels, and a valid conundrum.

Especially since May 2017, Jeff Sessions asked congressional leaders to repeal the Rohrabacher-Farr amendment, just so the Justice Department can withhold federal funds from those states that legalized cannabis on any level, including medical use.

On January 4th, 2018, Sessions rescinded the 'Cole Memorandum' which had prevented federal prosecutors from bringing charges against state legalized marijuana use, any sales person telling you that any CBD, hemp, or cannabis product 'is legal' is 100% lying, wrong, and either knowingly full of crap or willing to gamble on the odds.

So, because of these legal differences, and political winds of change, there are potentially even greater concerns that could impact every American. Understand, there are still some major (and real) concerns regarding the various types of insurance, liability, and even employment.

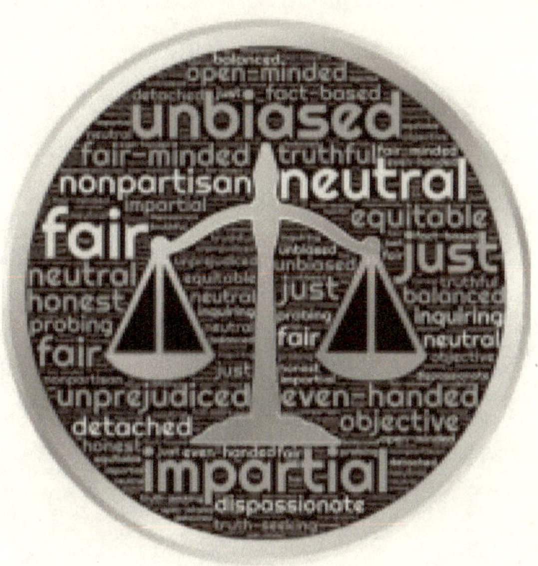

INSURANCE AND BENEFIT CONCERNS

1. WORKERS COMP -

When you could get hurt, are involved in, or cause an insurance claim, causing or are a party to, any accident that could harm yourself, or either another person or valuable property, YOU will likely be required to have blood and urine test for drugs and alcohol.

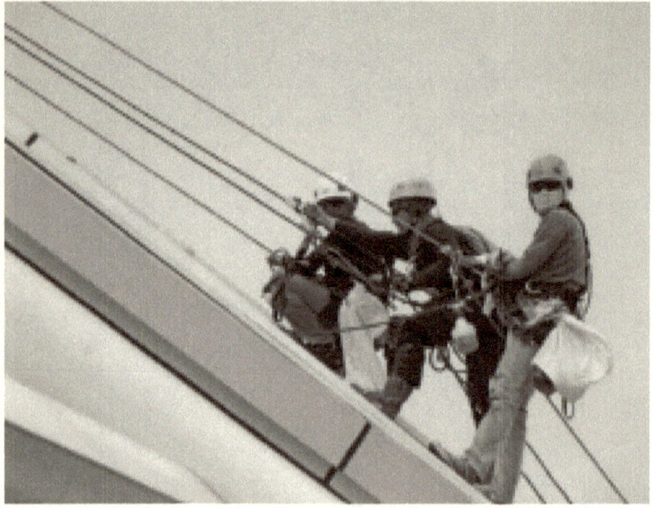

As of today, any THC found, even in legal states, COULD prohibit you from getting coverage or benefits... job insurance, loss wage protections, or any disability claims gone forever.

So far, only five states—Connecticut, Maine, Minnesota, New Jersey and New Mexico—officially require insurers to pay workers comp claims involving medical marijuana use; and even then it's not a 100% guarantee, depending on the job, the situation, and the level of THC in the system.

Example: Once evidence showed THC in a man's system, even though it wasn't believed to be related to the cause of the accident or injury, WCC denied his claims, and refused to pay his medical bills, time off work, retaining, and other costs. The reason: Oklahoma workers' comp law siting the fact he broke Federal Drug Laws by having THC in his system.

2. INSURANCE CLAIMS: -

While it's been pointed out that insurance covers the stupid, and accidental accidents... however, it does not cover the guilty in criminal acts, like driving drunk or under the influence of drugs. Those choices could cost you, personally.

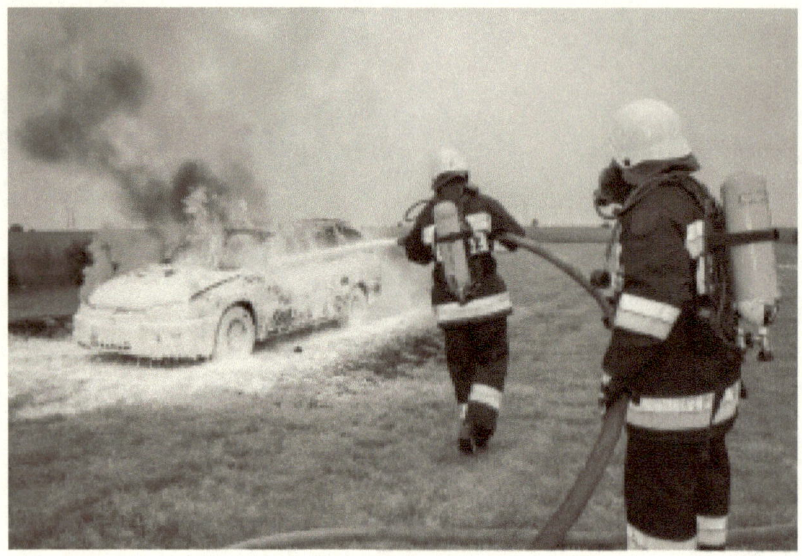

Insurers, in many states, are allowed to deny certain claims – in all or part – if alcohol or drugs are shown to be involved in the accident or action that caused the claim. Particularly if the claimant(s) are the ones intoxicated. "Wherever you're 'in public' – off your own property, especially.

You need to understand the statutes and state laws that apply, so that you are aware of the consequences of your actions.

3. LIFE INSURANCE CLAIMS –

Be aware of the exclusions list, because right now, nearly every policy has an over generalized exclusion of 'any illegal drugs.'

Marijuana Businessman Denied Derek Peterson, CEO of Terra Tech Corp, Life Insurance by Mutual of Omaha on June 13th 2016. Their letter stated, "we cannot accept premium(s) from individuals or entities who are associated with the marijuana industry."

While many policies will merely charge a higher rate for marijuana users, and honor the policy (if disclosed). However, there have been some dispute cases (after autopsy), where the insurance company claims "Material Misrepresentations on the Application.' A few families have hired attorneys and won; most have lost.

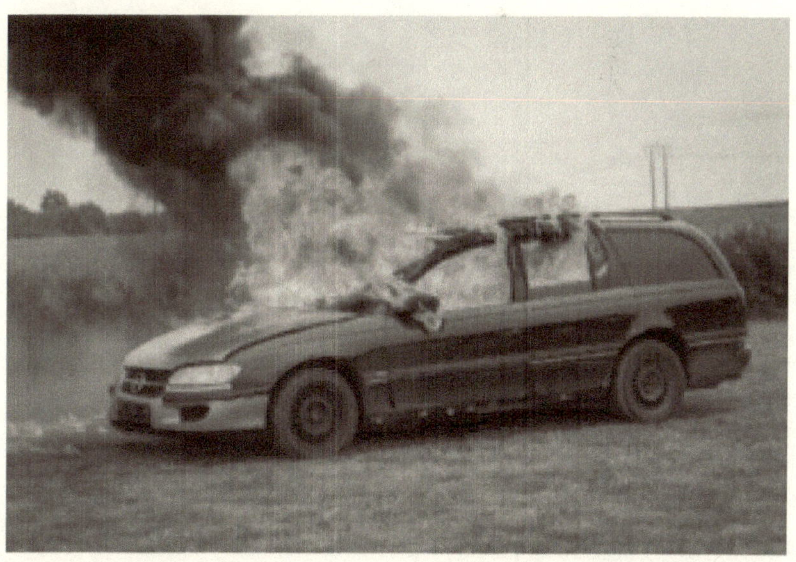

Whenever there is a question on a life insurance application you should be honest, and fully disclosed.

It is better they turn you down, or raise the premiums, than to have your loved ones thinking everything is 'in order' only to fight about things after the fact. Life insurance companies are not required by law to either report or investigate when they issue a policy, they usually take an applicant's answers as true.

If there are questions, check with an attorney to be sure of what the rules are now. Federal and State Group Life Insurance Claims are often controlled by federal statutes.

4. MALPRACTICE INSURANCE –

Talk about a wild double edge sword. Real Licensed Physicians are currently banned from 'prescribing' any cannabis product that aren't specifically FDA approved,

If they do, and are caught, they could lose their license to practice medicine, even in states that allow recreational or medical marijuana use. That is because it is clearly, and still, against federal law.

While they cannot 'prescribe' it, like they would other medicines; some have found what they believe is a legal loop hole, based on semantics: depending upon the individual state laws, and the regulations within their profession and specialty (which each doctor needs to verify for themselves – with their own attorney and licensing board) some believe they can 'suggest' or 'recommend' or 'certify' a cannabis product... in some states; IF they determine their patient *might* likely qualify for its use and may benefit, based on science. Doctors that are NOT prescribing should be sure to let their insurance provider know that, as it could lower your premium costs... **All that has a direct impact on INSURANCE companies, which often seek any excuse or reason they can to deny paying out.**

Most people hearing 'insurance' think about 'health insurance,' which is important, but there are really a variety of insurance types, as you've seen (in this section). However, there is another indirect impact: MALPRACTICE Insurance. That pesky major expense every doctor has to have, if they really want to remain in business.

However, the Malpractice Insurance Providers WILL NOT COVER ANY CASE where a licensed physician RECOMMENDS (suggests, or prescribes) any cannabis medication that is not specifically and implicitly FDA & DEA approved. Because of that, an Ohio based company, Cannasure, cropped up, hoping to fill the gap in some states. (Again, the doctor's need to check with their own legal counsel and licensing rules and regulations. Cannasure hopes to become a supplemental option.

5. HOME OWNERS INSURANCE –

A federal court in Hawaii ruled in 2012 that a homeowner's policy did NOT cover the theft of her marijuana plants grown for medicinal use. Neither would fire, volcano, nor flood insurance. Unless you have an addendum, or rider, that specifically states your cannabis (plant(s), product, or stash) are specifically covered, you can bet they absolutely will not be covered, replaced, or valued for any repayment in the event of any loss or claim. You are on your own.

The insurance company in the above example was USAA. They argued that because marijuana is federally classified as an illegal Schedule I substance (akin to heroin, morphine, and LSD) they were under no obligation to cover the loss at all. The court ultimately agreed with USAA, stating that even though Hawaii law permits the use of marijuana for medicinal use it is illegal under the Controlled Substances Act and therefore not subject to homeowners' insurance coverage.

There have been similar reports from other states also. It seems the most common claimed cases have been:

> - Burglary - someone stealing marijuana (plants or product)
> - Loss of plants/product destroyed in fire, flood, natural disaster

Further, IF the 'cannabis' can be determined to be the CAUSE, or the insurance company can claim 'criminal enterprise' – it is also possible they can try to deny THE ENTIRE CLAIM, in the event there were other losses (like your home burns down). If that happens, you are only hope is getting an attorney… and fighting it in court, which will take more time and money. With no guarantee of results.

Again, ASK your insurance provider, and make sure you **GET APPROVALS IN WRITING (and secure those documents off site).** If it is already in writing, and you are within the compliance boundaries, there should not be a problem.

6. INSURANCE POLICY LEGALESE –

Different companies have different wording, but nearly every policy we have ever seen and heard of, regardless what the company is insuring, tends to have loop holes, exceptions, and ways they can limit or deny claims. Sometimes the wording is specific: "any act, case, or proof of suicide removes all liability by Company xyz, and terminates policy with prejudice, without any payout." (or similar terminology).

Other policies might have something more cryptic, like:- "Company xyz's damages shall not include, or cover, any civil or criminal fines, sanctions, penalties or forfeitures, actions, or criminal acts, whether or not related to, or as a result of local, state, or federal regulations, statutes, ordinance, laws, or rules of civil or criminal procedure, and/or any such judgments." That's a mouth full. But, if you're looking for coverage… agreeing to those type of words is out. Because they will not have to pay you a dime, and even if you try to sue them.

There is another concern, which is even potentially more scary than just not getting paid, or getting your property replaced, and that is a 'hold-harmless' clause that redirects back to the insured (cough, YOU – if you have a claim through a policy with them). That allows them to *maybe* pay a third party, but then come after you for any payouts, costs associated with the payout or collections, if for no other reason than they can, and will at least get money or a 'write off.'

"Dishonest, deliberate, intentionally wrongful, fraudulent, malicious acts **or omissions, or criminal**, committed by or at the direction of, including but not limited to with the knowledge of, or ratified, **by any Insured**."

If you're in an auto accident, your house burns down, you're involved in a work place accident, someone sues you because of your job/action… you might well be all on your own… without any policy or umbrella protecting you or limiting your liability. As with all contracts, it is THE WORDING YOU AGREED TO.

7. VA (VETERAN'S AFFAIRS) AND DRUG TESTING –

Aside from the potential loss of VA Benefits if the wrong persons chooses to make an issue of any THC found in the blood stream, derived from unapproved consumption. This only impacts the Veterans actually getting VA Benefits or using the VA Hospitals. **Some VA officials have chosen to 'look the other way' particularly if PTSD, chronic pain management is required, or any neurological issues exist.** As of 20 September 2018, on their web site, www.publichealth.va.gov/marijuana.asp, the following is clearly stated:

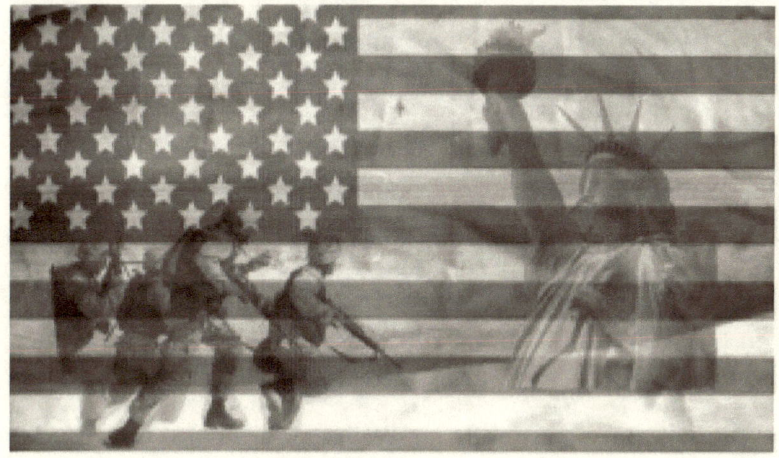

"Several states in the U.S. have approved the use of marijuana for medical and/or recreational use. Veterans should know that federal law classifies marijuana – including all derivative products of cannabis sativa – are still a Schedule One controlled substance. This makes it illegal in the eyes of the federal government.

The U.S. Department of Veterans Affairs is required to follow all federal laws including those regarding marijuana. As long as the Food and Drug Administration classifies marijuana as Schedule One VA health care providers may not recommend it or assist Veterans to obtain it.

Veteran participation in state marijuana programs does not affect eligibility for VA care and services. VA providers can and do discuss marijuana use with Veterans as part of comprehensive care planning, and adjust treatment plans as necessary.

Some things Veteran need to know about marijuana and the VA:
- will not be denied VA benefits because of marijuana use.
- are encouraged to discuss marijuana use with their VA providers.
- health care providers will record marijuana use in the Veteran's medical record in order to have the information available in treatment planning. As with all clinical information, this is part of the confidential medical record and protected under patient privacy and confidentiality laws.
- clinicians may not recommend medical marijuana.
- **clinicians may only prescribe medications that have been approved by the FDA** for medical use. At present most products containing Tetrahydrocannabinol (THC), Cannabidiol (CBD), or other cannabinoids are not approved for this purpose.
- clinicians may not complete paperwork/forms required for Vet patients to participate in state-approved marijuana programs.
- pharmacies may not fill prescriptions for medical marijuana.
- will not pay for medical marijuana prescriptions from any source.
- scientists may conduct research on marijuana benefits and risks,

and potential for abuse, under regulatory approval. Please address questions related to research to: VHABLRD-CSRD@va.gov

- The use or possession of marijuana is prohibited at all VA medical centers, locations and grounds. When you are on VA grounds it is federal law that is in force, not the laws of the state.

- Veterans who are VA employees are subject to drug testing under the terms of employment.

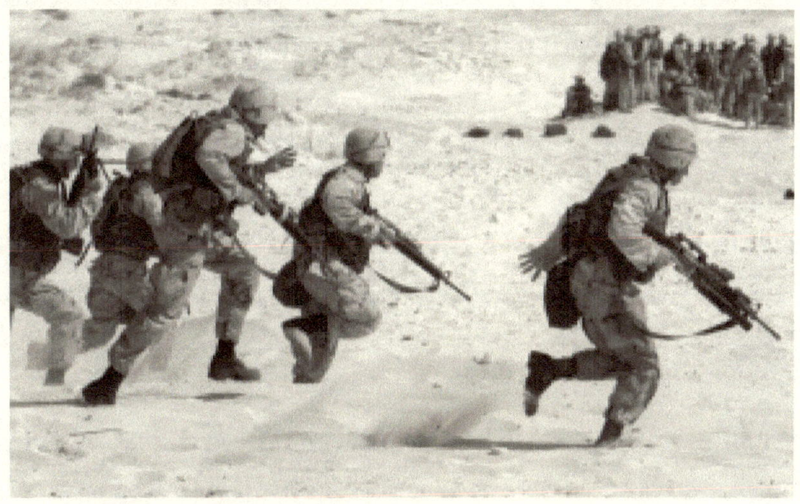

Caution is still given, because **rules are always subject to change**, but once things are IN YOUR RECORD, it will not be easily or inexpensively removed. If politicians, the DEA or FDA, or any branch of the military choose to tighten up because of some policy changes, it will only take one wrong person to make life more challenging. I am not saying to lie.

I am saying BE CAREFUL and AWARE! It could become a lifetime of denial of benefits.

According to the VA web site, and many of the doctors have spoken out, FOR certain ailments they are treating, which THC or CBD has shown to positively effect. They are advocating for their patients, and looking the other way as necessary, and becoming more tolerant, and aware. However, **they are clear, IT IS STILL AGAINST FEDERAL LAW**, and their tolerance does not change that fact.

Considering the VA cut millions of veterans off prescriptions for chronic pain management in 2015 without warning, anything is possible.

President Trump signed an Executive Order allowing 'experimental drugs' to be used (by the general public) right after the VA forced hundreds of thousands of Veterans to cold turkey off their chronic pain meds; however, that Executive Order had nothing to do with CBD, cannabis, or Veterans.

Cutting the Veterans off their chronic pain management necessarily increased veterans self-medicating with alcohol. Cannabis, or other 'street drugs.' Some Vets were offered alternatives, like acupuncture or chiropractors, muscle relaxers, or anti- inflammatory drugs; but not all that had been getting pain killers and certain other discontinued drugs to treat chronic problems, were given effective alternatives.

The VA tests for everything, all illegal drugs, as well as levels of those prescription drugs the veteran is supposed to be on to verify they are really taking them. So DO NOT LIE! Some of the VA hospitals are not testing as strictly for THC content, especially if they think there is a reason it is used by the veteran...

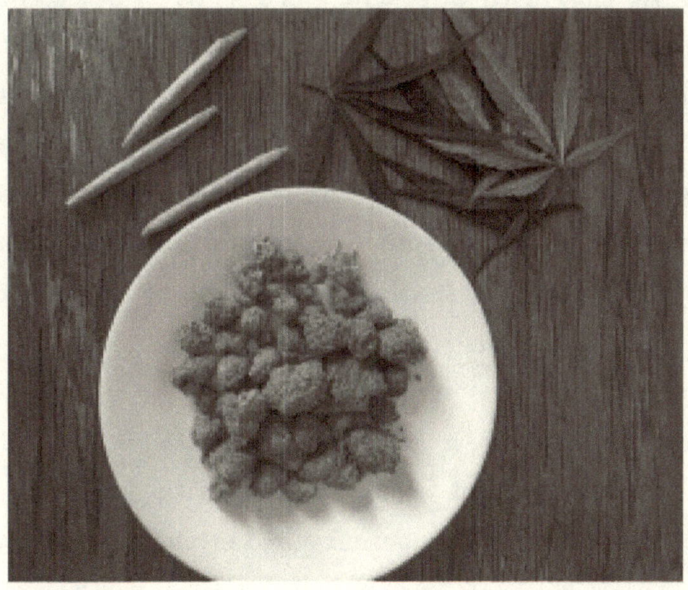

The winds of change seem to happen at the whim or the National Budget and who ever happens to be in the White House. Personally, I wouldn't bet anyone's continued VA benefits on what the VA is doing, or the thoroughness of the third party test requested, often with little notice (if you regularly use the VA Hospital for your medical care). **Be careful**.

Would you take a chance?

I will tell you what I told my family members & friends that go to the VA for healthcare services: BE CAREFUL! Especially if you live in a state it's not clearly legal, until and unless the VA officially approves it; UNLESS you are otherwise dying within the next 6 to 12 months, or suffering in a way the VA just isn't able to help you with. As a Veteran with an Honorable Discharge, you get VA Entitlements or Tri-Care, because of your Service to Our Country.

However, those things are paid for with a budget politicians often try to manipulate, and cut costs in one place so they can spend all that (and usually more) in another place. To most of those politicians, the veterans are fodder, a number, to be used how they see fit. If they are trying to cut some of the defense budget, anything is possible. Another words, most politicians, especially those that never served in any branch of the military or a military school, cannot really be trusted to support the military, or aging veterans, any further than you can throw them.

If someone at the VA approves it, try to get THEIR APPROVAL in WRITING if you can! Ultimately it could be your word against someone's, if they could die, get transferred, or relocated. The new person that replaces them might not be as accepting. **Guess who wins if there is a dispute.**

If you are a veteran, COPY THE PAGE ON THEIR WEBSITE (screen capture from September 20th, 2018, and links, are at the end of reference section). **TALK TO YOUR DOCTOR about it, and how it may (or may not) help you.** Remember, NEVER EVER set foot on federal property with any non-prescription drug or alcohol on your person, or in your vehicle! It IS ABSOLUTELY AGAINST FEDERAL LAW! The powers to be could be looking for excuses to kick people off the 'free programs' in some regions at a moment's notice; especially if the political winds shift… because of budget cuts or no reason at all. Especially when people have chronic issues which equate to chronic costs. It is important to think ahead, and talk to them before you do something… if at all possible. Remember, THC remains in the blood stream for up to 45 days. Good Luck, and Thank you for your service!

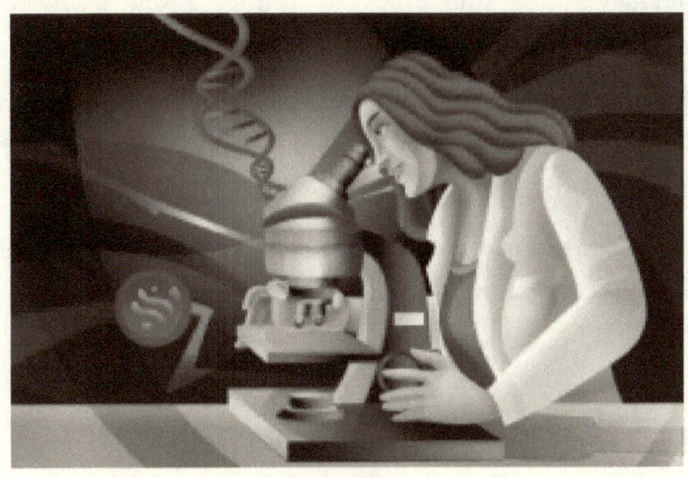

As the VA's requirements, and testing, are different from facility to facility, state to state, even doctor to doctor, it's important to be aware. In general, the Basic Policy in some state VA hospitals seems to be to look the other way. However, there are no guarantees that cannot (or will not) change without notice.

If your PCG (Primary Care Giver) does not have a problem with it you are good, but you should check with them. That said, it is still federal law so VA has to abide by it (as they want). That was what a High-Level VA Doctor said on the topic; different doctors may check and or not.

However, since the VA has stopped handing out the prescription pain killers as freely, frequently, and in the quantities it was... some facilities have seemingly lightened up on the use of quality CBD oils, and even THC found in the system. Especially since President Trumps, Executive Order authorizing experimental medication use.

There are quite a few promising studies, but the inconsistency between manufacturers and differences in batches (even from the same manufacturer) are wildly different, varied and real. It's our opinion, and observation, that there are way too many inconsistencies in the production and processing of CBD oil. Further, the reality is that it is still against Federal law, and state laws in 42 of the states (though it appears that is likely to change in many more states, and potentially federally within the next decade… rendering the legality issue moot).

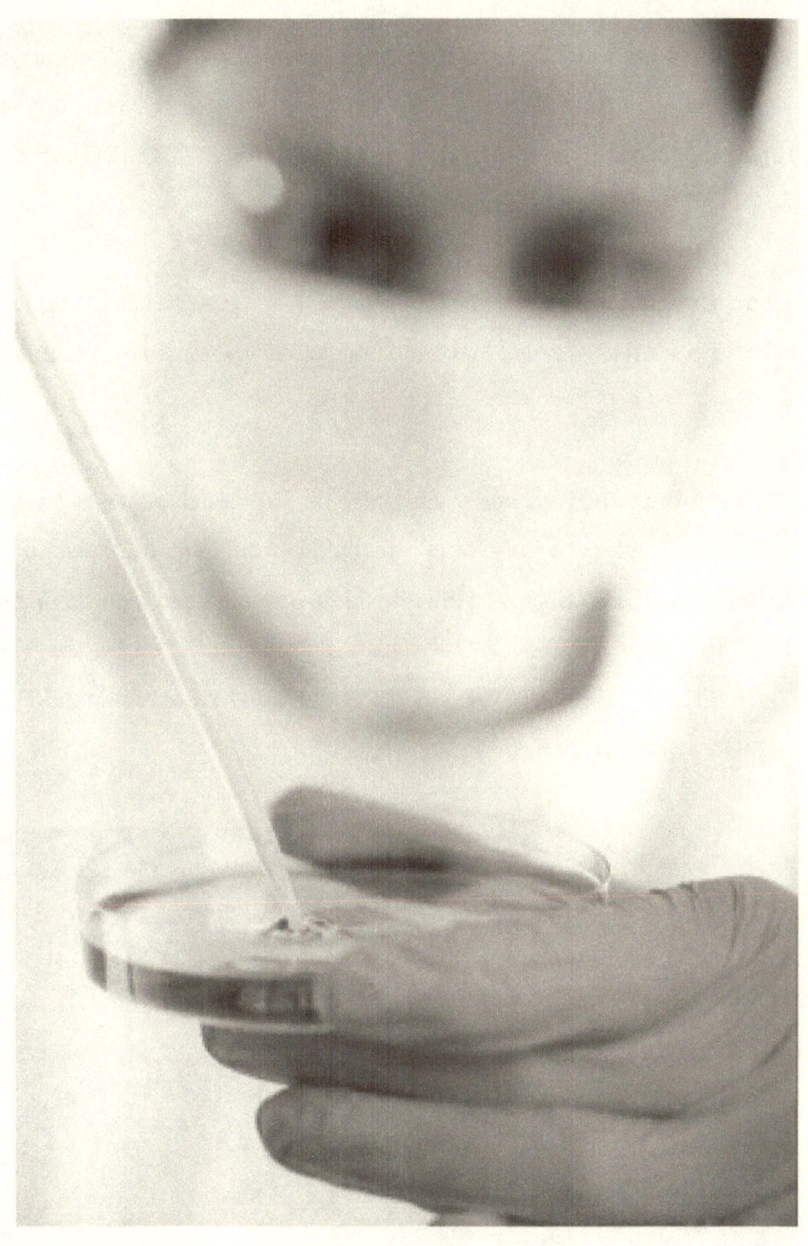

Federal law does not yet recognize medical marijuana, or really offer any legal approval for CBD Oils. All cannabis related products are still regulated through the Controlled Substances Act (CSA) (21 U.S.C. § 811).

Under the Act, every controlled substance is categorized according to its relative potential for abuse and medicinal value, and danger to the general public.

The CSA does NOT currently recognize the difference between medical and recreational use of any 'drug' - including marijuana, marijuana treats (edibles), or CBD Oils... and the federal government can treat them each like all other controlled substances, until and unless they are SPECIFICALLY FDA & DEA APPROVED, and comply with all FDA regulations! Awareness is key!

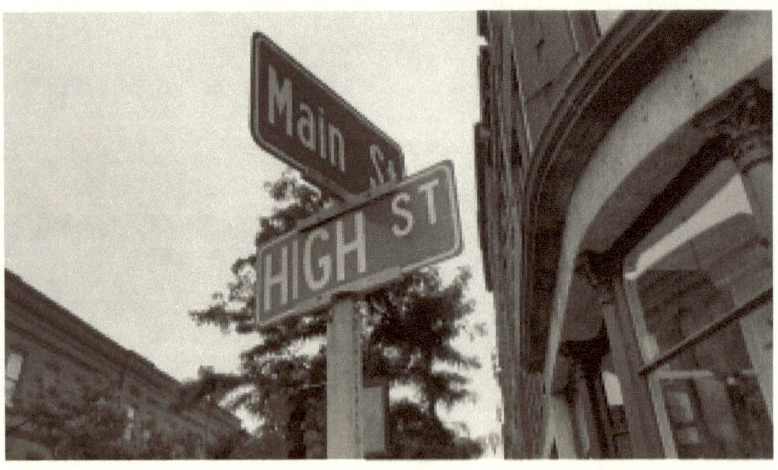

Under the CSA, marijuana is still classified as a Schedule I drug, or "highly addictive and having no medical value." The ONLY *maybe* exception would be for those people officially taking one of the FDA approved PRESCRIPTION DRUGS, which contain some level of THC.

On September 28th 2018, the DEA put the FDA 'approved' cannabis drugs 'with CBD' in a SCHEDULE V listing, which it defines as having the lowest potential for abuse, such as drugs used to treat diarrhea and cough suppressants, under the CSA. The DEA action means that GW Pharmaceuticals can sell Epidiolex, a treatment for pediatric epilepsy, but did not go further to reclassify CBD as a whole.

WHY MD'S CHOICE DOES NOT SELL IT:

MD's Choice, is focused on nutrition, since 1995. Over the last five years, we were bombarded with 'offers' to add CBD Oil to our line, but purposefully haven't, and won't, unless it's 100% legal by state **and federal laws**; probably not even then.

We had greater opportunity to look deeper into CBD Oil and cannabis than most people, because of our involvement in the industry, to see more of the actual scientific findings, behind the scenes. We believe it is important to acknowledge what the science shows it can actually do, as well as what is can NOT do; and discuss the real world limits.

CBD Oil focuses on NERVES, and interacts with the brain and spinal column. It has shown promise for treating certain types of Epilepsies, to the point the FDA has officially approved a 'drug' product made of 99.7% CBD as the primary active ingredient for the treatment of epilepsy.

FDA approval does not guarantee 'it works' in any fashion, or that it's necessarily even safe... however, their approval does guarantee some more (and likely better) research, closer evaluation and scrutiny, and the reality of an opportunity to do well for some specific ailments.

It's more likely to list known side-effects, including (for some drugs) that *might* cause feeling that lead to a variety of serious issues, such as anal leakage, liver damage, and even homicide, suicide, or even death.

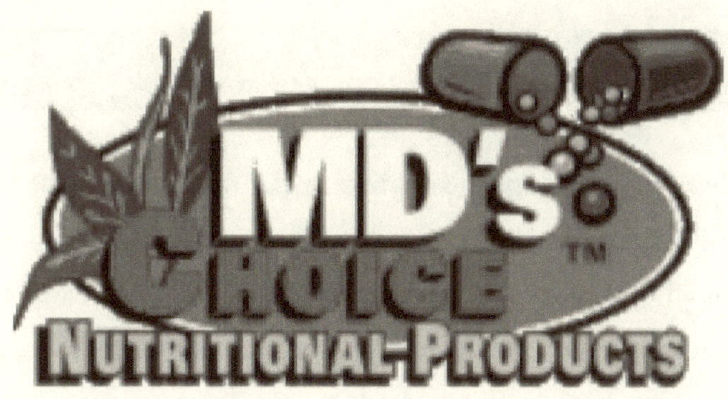

MD's Choice spent more than 20 years focused on two primary goals:

1) trying to help spread ethical & scientific education of others on the topics of health & nutrition, as well as

2) to design and distribute quality supplements targeting specific ailments (joints, digestion, reproduction, and general health) that actually helps in the right way – by supplying the body the nutrients it needs, in forms it can readily use, to assist the body in healing itself when possible.

MD's Choice absolutely understands the benefits of medicine, quality, process, consistency, purification, production, and usefulness. We strive to pay attention to things that can improve health, quality and longevity of life; and will attempt to share that information with others, as it becomes available. For more information check out www.mdchoice.com for the people products, and www.VetSupplements.com for animal product information and a variety of articles and links.

HOW IT All STARTED (Some History)

It is always tough to figure out where to 'put' the history, at the beginning where it technically belongs, or toward the end, because most people don't care, or will just skim over it, or ignore it altogether. We chose the latter, because some may find it interesting, and learn a few things they just did not previously know (and frankly, I thought it was interesting. Stuff most people do not know, realizes, or remember).

Since much of this information was 'new to us' prior to the research for this publication, we believed it would be helpful to understand a bit of the history that has led up to where things are – legally – RIGHT NOW. We believe it will also help you understand some of the directions things are likely to go in the next three to eight years, as more science is released… and more facts become publicly known, and more states push for legalization. Things really have come a long way.

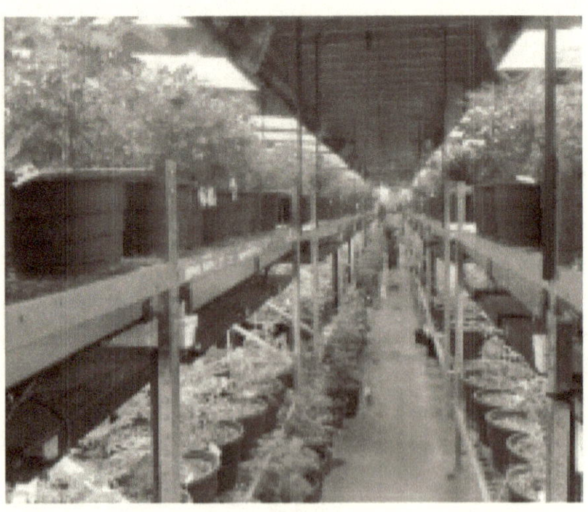

In 1963 a young organic chemist, in Israel, named Raphael Mechoulam, who was working at the Weizmann Institute of Science outside Tel Aviv, decided to 'officially' do some research into the actual chemical composition of cannabis plants. He thought it was odd that morphine could be derived from opium back in 1805, and cocaine harvested from coca leaves in 1855, yet scientists had no idea what the principal psychoactive ingredient in marijuana really were.

"It was just a plant, with a mélange of unidentified compounds." says Mechoulam, in 2017, at age 84.

So Mechoulam went through the government channels, contacting the Israeli national police with his plan. They released five kilos of confiscated Lebanese hashish to him, to get the ball rolling.

Within a few weeks, he and his research group isolated an array of substances, which he injected separately into rhesus monkeys. Only one of those chemicals had any quick observable effect. "Normally the rhesus monkey is quite an aggressive individual," he says. But when injected with this compound (later named tetrahydrocannabinol, THC), the monkeys became emphatically calm. "Sedated, I would say," he recalls with a chuckle.

Further testing isolated the compound further, as the plant's principal active ingredient, THC. The mind-altering essence that makes people 'high.'

Mechoulam, along with a colleague, officially discovered THC, and elucidated the chemical structure of cannabidiol (CBD), another key ingredient in marijuana. CBD has become the basis for turning opinions, because of many medical uses since proven, with no psychoactive effect on humans.

Mechoulam is a respected member of the Israel Academy of Sciences and Humanities, and an emeritus professor at Hebrew University's Hadassah Medical School, where he still runs a lab. He has authored more than 420 scientific papers, holds 25 patents, and has spent a lifetime studying cannabis. A plant he calls a "medicinal treasure trove waiting to be discovered." Marijuana was growing in popularity for recreational use, particularly among those who were youth in the 60's & 70's. Since it was directly competing with the same 'customers' the alcohol industry was targeting, one of the world's best marketing campaign started; quietly cheered, in the background, by Big Pharma (the drug companies) and Tabaco companies, both of which were busy filing patents for cannabis related products, uses, and formulas.

If you doubt, look up Patent 6630507, it is the US GOVERNMENT PATENT, granted to the Department of Health and Human Services in 2003. The NIH (National Institutes of Health) uncovered potential innovations, so they applied for the patent. Supposedly, it allows them to control some of the research, and allow others (on THEIR approved list) to do testing and research.

Scientists with the NIH were searching for antioxidant qualities, when they first applied for the patent in 1999. Interestingly, it ONLY covers SOME non-psychoactive compounds found in the plant to protect the brain from damage or degeneration caused by certain diseases, such as cirrhosis." The patent also states, "No signs of toxicity or serious side effects have been observed following chronic administration of cannabidiol to healthy volunteers, even in large acute doses...." Which means that, in 1999, the government officials admitted to knowing that certain compounds in cannabis have medicinal properties, and just as importantly, those compounds are safe for human consumption. The abstract they included stated that cannabinoids act as antioxidants, which were thought to effective in the treatment of Alzheimer's, Parkinson's, and HIV dementia

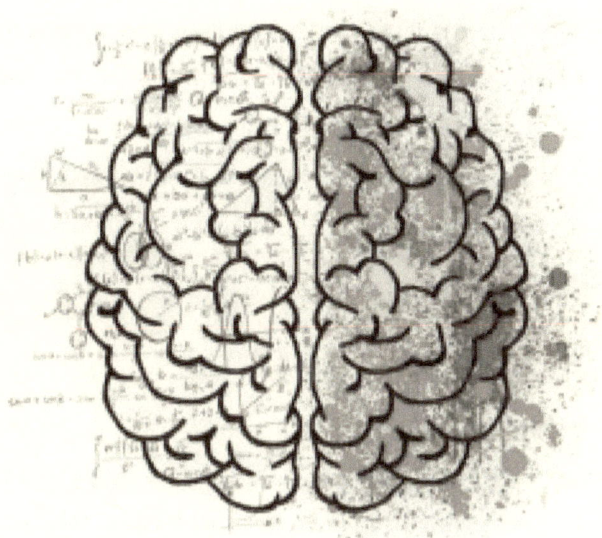

"THE WAR ON DRUGS." If you cannot control it, ban it. If you cannot collect taxes from it, outlaw it. The patent, mentioned above, not only proves that there are at least some serious medicinal properties possible with cannabis, but that the government has known about it for decades. You see, Patent 6,630,507 actually references 12 additional U.S. patents related to cannabis, dating back to 1942.

The concept and actions were easy for those lobbying against 'pot' (marijuana, weed, THC, etc.). The government was coming out of prohibition on alcohol, and needed a new enemy. Marijuana and heroin were the easy targets, those deadly and addictive opioids; or so they claimed, as they lumped them all together in the creation of laws, bans, and criminal sentencing guidelines. Laws were selectively applied, both geographically and income wise, the poor were imprisoned or ignored, the middle class fined or jailed, and the rich... well, they slipped through with technicalities.

Since it was tough for the government to tax and control, laws were created. Growing pot is far easier than making your own alcohol, so the war was on. The government found it was easier to 'outlaw' cannabis than to establish and enforce existing rules & laws. Easier to ban, than establish and enforce rules for public intoxication that could endanger others. Easier to blanket outlaw than have regulations for commercial growing and reselling.

Many blame the alcohol industry, because they did not want the competition (for intoxicating effects); and the other industries that knew they would profit for many years over the 'War on Drugs' and what it was projected to cost the American taxpayers, and mean to their industry.

Yes, some of the biggest Big Pharma (commercial drug manufacturers), because they did not want the competition either. It quickly became easier when someone(s), somewhere, started 'lacing' the marijuana with 'PCP' (angel dust), and LSD, and young people started experiencing 'trips' and hallucinations, and people started to really get hurt. Laws were pushed through to 'save the kids' – the younger generation that just doesn't know any better. It was a quick push in many geographies, because the 'tainted' marijuana was real, and bad trips were caught on camera and in the media. There was also a vast difference in quality, potency, and potential safety of the 'raw material.'

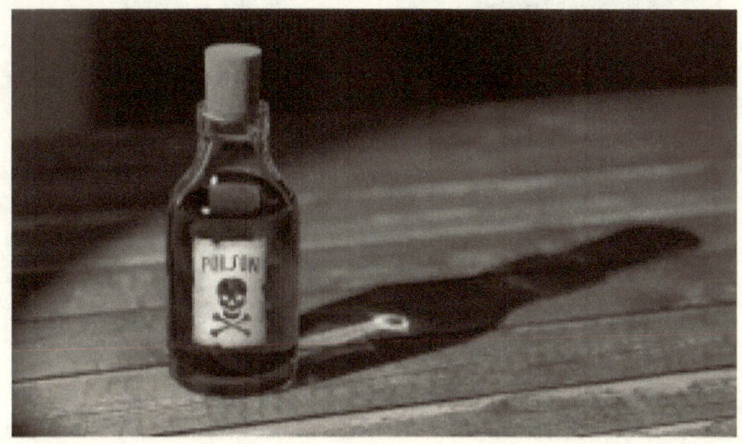

Remember, unless it's a matter of acute alcohol poisoning or a drunk driving type accident, alcohol abuse takes many years to cause enough harm to end a life, and is rarely blamed for shortening the life (even when the liver damage is obvious). Those 'bad trips' were causing problems within minutes or hours, and if the afflicted person survived, it was unknown what the affect would be on their life, long term.

Many believe politics pushed the federal agencies, FDA, DEA, and IRS to justify the ban, because pot (aka marijuana, weed, cannabis, etc.) could not easily be taxed or controlled since it could be grown in your home, your garden, in fields, and even the wild. There was no way to guarantee it could be kept out of the hands of young children, so fear was instilled; blaming conservatives for pushing the laws.

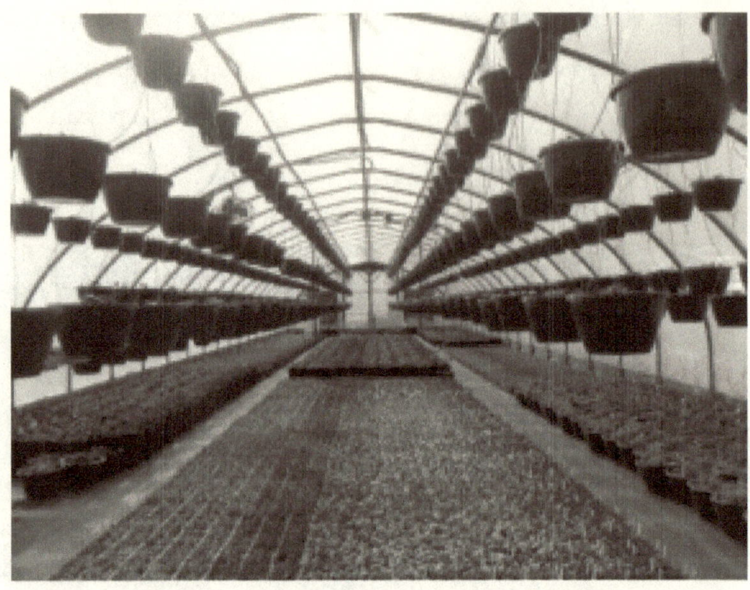

Since it has become partially legalized to treat children with interactive epilepsy… after tens of millions of people saw the before and after videos of the children having multiple seizures a day, and just how much it could really (visually to even strangers, and cameras) help those poor suffering children. States started pushing for at least some medical use laws, and removal of the restrictions. Yes, some children use it for medical reasons.

Just like the prohibition against alcohol at the turn of the century, cannabis has been demonized, propagandized, condemned, and outright lied about.

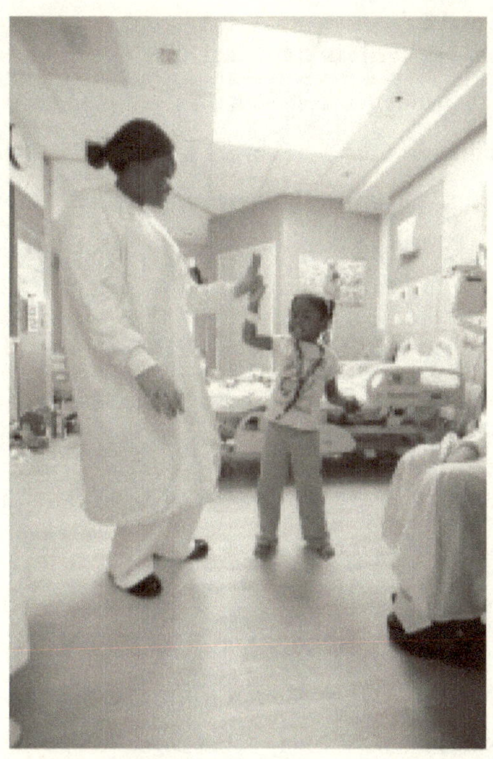

However, the reality is, today ALL cannabis, and related products, are still listed as a 'Schedule 1 Agent' (aka Narcotic: 'a drug with a high potential for abuse, and no currently accepted medical use') by the American Federal Government, and a few other governments around the world. Sadly, that label is disingenuous, especially when you consider the fact there really are a few hundred years of science, decades of actual 'peer reviewed' studies, and the FDA has officially approved a few forms, processes, and uses for medical purposes (for 'Big Pharma'). It is all about CONTROL and MONEY. Just imagine…

8,000 BC CHINESE records dating back to (in Taiwan to be specific) for assorted uses of hemp. It deals with using hemp for building materials, clothing, shoes, as well as medicinal use. Descriptions written in the world's oldest pharmacopoeia "Pen Ts'ao Ching" (written first century AD), suggest ancient Chinese cultures recognized benefits of hemp, and was also the first record to differentiate between 'industrial hemp' and 'marijuana' (male vs female plants… 'Industrial' vs 'medicinal' uses).

2,737L BC , FIRST MEDICAL USE DOCUMENTED, in specific references and directions of the Emperor Shen-Nung, who used specific parts of the female plant to make teas for medical use, as a natural pain treatment; as well as a topical, to apply as a poultice or ointment for rashes and irritation.

BETWEEN 2,000 AND 800 BC IN HINDU TEXT "ATHARVAVEDA," (exact date is disputed). Hemp was described as one of the '5 sacred plants.' Along about the same time period, ancient text was found, written by the Egyptian's, demonstrating hemp oil was an ingredient for eyewash. All that rolls back some serious history, and effective use throughout the centuries.

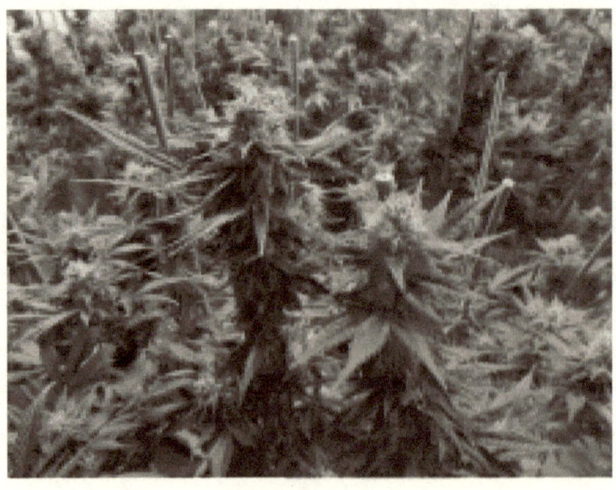

1616, FIRST CROP was documented on North America, it has been grown and used for a wide variety of things. At one point, the Virginia Assembly established laws that REQUIRED ALL CITIZENS to grow hemp.

1776, THE PLANT WAS ACCEPTED AS LEGAL TENDER in Maryland, Pennsylvania, Virginia, and Kentucky.

1800, EVERY STATE OF THE NEWLY FORMED UNITED STATES, was actively growing industrial hemp on huge scales.

1851, THE THIRD EDITION OF THE US PHARMACOPEIA, listed hemp extract among its medicines.

1906, "PURE FOOD AND DRUG ACT" (Start of the FDA), was enacted by President Theodore Roosevelt. The goal was well meaning: "to ban foreign and interstate trafficking of adulterated or mislabeled food and drug products." To establish some safety guidelines, 'to protect the people,' so they claimed. It specifically listed 'non-medical cannabis' as a poisonous drug. Many did not agree, even within the government. If you are curious, look up the 1914 'Hemp Note' – actual Federal Reserve Currency, depicting hemp cultivation here in America. The design of that **1913 FEDERAL RESERVE NOTE** (aka ten dollar bill) was printed, despite California, passing a law prohibiting the use of marijuana.

The California State Board of Pharmacy sponsored the law, banning marijuana, thinking they could target Mexicans living in the Los Angeles area, to either fine or imprison them OR to get them to leave the country.

1919, THE 18TH AMENDMENT WAS RATIFIED, banning the manufacture, transportation or sale of intoxicating liquors, ushering in the Prohibition Era. The same year, Congress passed the National Prohibition Act (also known as the Volstead Act), which offered guidelines on how to federally enforce Prohibition. Prohibition (for alcohol) lasted until December 1933, when the 21st Amendment was ratified, overturning the 18th. The question is how much did ALCOHOL industry have to do with taking out its competition, by pointing at drugs?

1930, THE FBN WAS CREATED; (FEDERAL BUREAU OF NARCOTICS) and at the height of the Great Depression, cannabis was blamed (for the Great Depression and influx of Mexicans entering American). That was used to create a war on drugs.

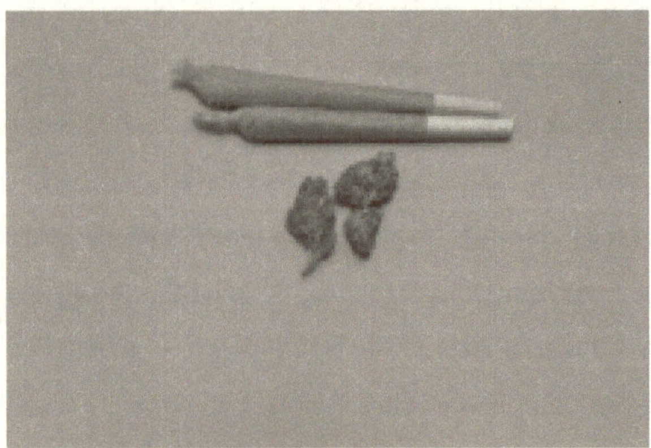

1936 FILM 'REEFER MADNESS' was released in an attempt to scare Americans into believing the plant was dangerous and the source of all societies' failures, and should be outlawed.

1937, MARIJUANA TAX ACT WENT INTO EFFECT, a year after the movie. It strictly regulated the cultivation and sale of all cannabis varieties, including 'hemp.' The government imposed a tax levy of $1 per ounce for medicinal use, and $100 per ounce for nonmedical use (remember, those were 1937 prices: when gasoline was just $0.10 a gallon, a brand new house cost under $5,000m and the top of the line new car could be had for under $800). It has been reported that the witness list for the hearings contained no one that had actually done any significant research into the effects of cannabis, it was all 'lynch mob' style voting based on emotion.

Mr. Anslinger, commissioner of the FBN, and led fear monger, testified that 'even a single marijuana cigarette could induce a homicidal mania, prompting people to want to kill those they love.' The bill passed, Roosevelt signed it into law. Clearly, the Act was only a means to keep marijuana out of the hands of poor people, and minorities, who might otherwise use alcohol. It was also to create both fines and control (court processes & sentencing) for those caught in possession (growing or using) 'the non-taxed drug.'

1937, AMA OPPOSED THE ACT, but were not on the witness list. The AMA (American Medical Association) firmly believed the Act would absolutely impede further research into medicinal worth of cannabis products. But it was pushed through congress anyhow, and became 'the law or the land.'

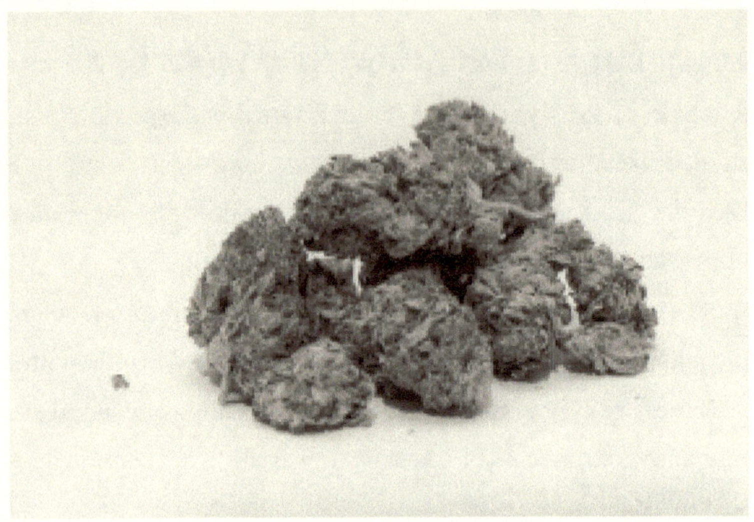

By now, the government is trying to scare the youth away, promote the anti-drug crusade, and gain adult support from their law.

1949, FEDERAL BUREAU OF NARCOTICS, in conjunction with the US Treasury, approved the film "SHE SHOULDA SAID NO!" produced to capitalize on the arrests of Lila Leeds and mega movie star Robert Mitchum on a charge of 'felony narcotics possession.' Note: Leeds was sentenced to 6 months in prison, with five years of probation, and basically black-balled from Hollywood. Then RKO studio chief, Howard Hughes, assembled a team of lawyers to defend Mitchum, who did his 6 months, and silently went back to work in the movie industry on a variety of Hughes projects. His record did not destroy his career, but he was never the same again. This exploitation film followed in the spirit of other propaganda films such as the 1936 films Reefer Madness and Marihuana, attempting to 'scare' people from smoking Cannabis.

1951 ANTI-MARIJUANA PROPAGANDA FILM, "The Terrible Truth" where they claim marijuana leads to intravenous heroin use, crime and prostitution. Total scare tactics. Generally, all cannabis remained a 'controlled substance.'

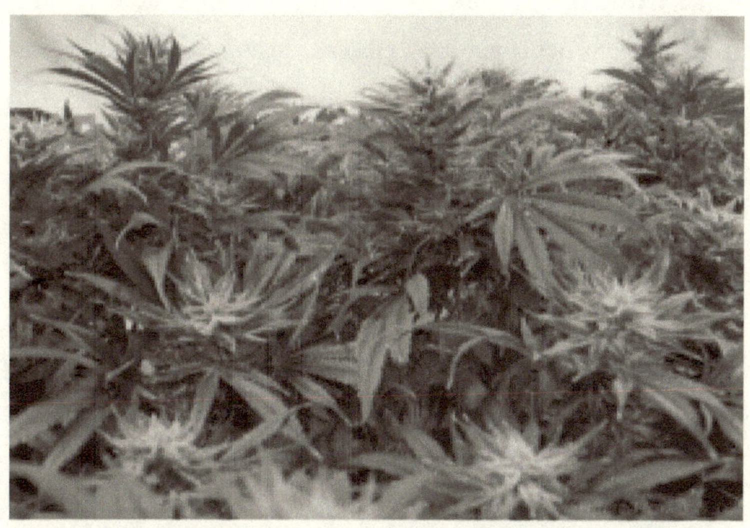

1951, DR. HARRIS ISBELL DISPUTED The 'Insanity, Crime, And Addiction Theories' telling Congress that "smoking marijuana has no unpleasant aftereffects, no dependence is developed on the drug, and the practice can easily be stopped at any time." Despite the professional testimony from the then Director of Research at the Public Health Service Hospital,, Congress pushed up the penalties on growers, sellers, and end users.

Many of the states followed the federal example, and states like Louisiana, for instance, created sentences ranging from 5 to 99 years, without parole or probation, for the sale or possession of narcotic drugs. (Including marijuana). Their rational was not that pot was deadly, highly addictive, or even promoted prostitution, burglary, robbery, and murder, as many against it had previously claimed, but that it was a "STEPPINGSTONE" to heroin or other hard, nasty, and destructive drugs.

For the most part, as long as laws and penalties were targeting the minorities and poor people, most citizens remained blissfully ignorant and silent; accepting heavy handed and unjust punitive approaches of the lengthy sentences for non-violent citizens; so long as it wasn't 'them' – or their child, brother, sister, parent, relatives they liked, or the person that signed their pay checks.

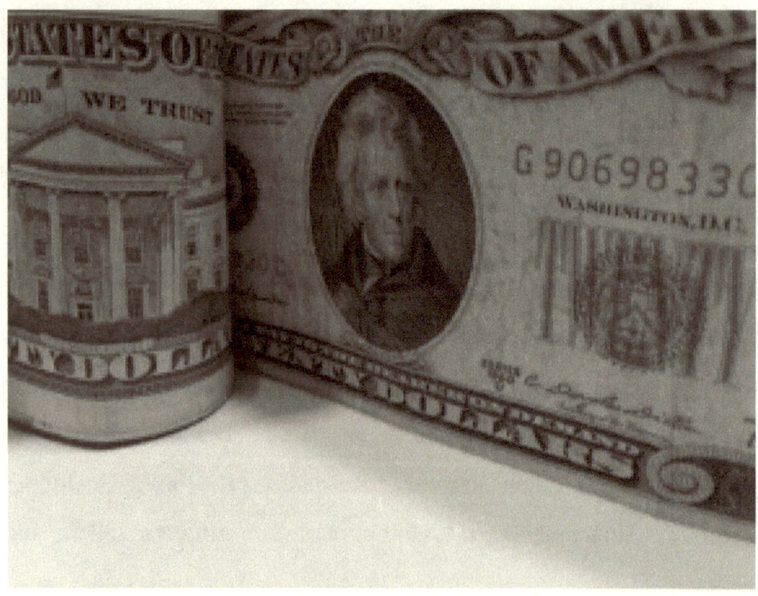

1955 TO 1975, VIET NAM WAR toward the end, an Estimated 30% of the US troops engaged in regular usage of marijuana; and, at home, weed made its way to the white college students, many of which were trying to avoid the draft. Seeing either war hero's or white lives ruined by the pot laws, with huge life ending sentences, softened public attitudes when it became their sons & daughters, their relatives, and their peers being locked away for far too many years.

1960'S MARIJUANA USE BECAME COMMON PLACE from the beginning of the 'hippy' movement, which pretty much started with the end of the Vietnam War. Weed, Pot, MaryJane, Marijuana, Smoke, became the topic of comedy, movies, and was safer than alcohol, which people could grow themselves. Marijuana had become 'the drug' for recreational use and an alternative to alcohol for most in the 'Peace & Love to All' crusade.

1970, RICHARD M. NIXON SIGNED IN THE CSA (CONTROLLED SUBSTANCES ACT) while many states softened on laws surrounding the use and possession of marijuana, the federal government pushed through that bill, making it a law. Which became stacks of regulations, new crimes, more fines, and stronger punishments; with exceptions only for the rich. It became a grand gesture, claiming to 'stop all drugs.'

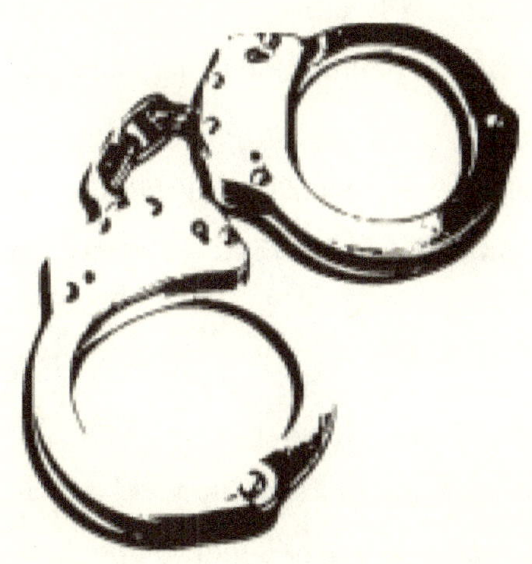

However, during a 1994 interview with John Ehrlichman, Nixon's domestic policy chief, who provided inside info stating that "The War on Drugs" campaign was initially designed to help Nixon keep his job. Ehrlichman was quoted as saying: "We knew we couldn't make it illegal to be either against the war or blacks, but by getting the public to associate the hippies with marijuana and blacks with heroin, and then criminalizing both heavily, we could disrupt those communities. We could arrest their leaders, raid their homes, break up their meetings, and vilify them night after night on the evening news. Did we know we were lying about the drugs? Of course, we did." Ehrlichman said.

1972 - 1977, 11 STATES DECRIMINALIZED MARIJUANA POSSESSION. Jimmy Carter ran on a political campaign to decriminalize marijuana, and won. Of course, he was a farmer… and understood the benefit of health crops, and growing profit… and the industrial use.

During Carter's first year, the Senate Judiciary Committee "voted to decriminalize up to one ounce of marijuana." This is one of the only positive things Carter really accomplished, and few people ever mention it today. This is particularly important, because it demonstrates just how much cannabis has been political fodder for decades!

It has been legal, and decriminalized BEFORE… and for most of our country's history. **Do not forget that… because it will likely CYCLE AGAIN!**

Most states ceased all new criminal actions with 'pot' – and did not seem to care about 'personal use' or 'home growers,' just large scale operations, and criminal enterprises. Some non-violent offenders were even released from prison & jail. But when Nixon left office, so did most of his anti-drug rhetoric, for a time. Soon after his resignation, to avoid impeachment, the War on Drugs took a slight hiatus.

1978, PCP (ANGEL DUST) BECAME ILLEGAL in the United States, because it was causing people to 'flip out' and hurt themselves, or others. It gave some Superman like strength, and many demonstrated suicidal tendencies, delusions of flight (until they hit the ground), or being some wild or huge animal (bear, bull, and horse have been reported as common delusions). When those results hit the college crowd, then general public became afraid.

Especially when 'little Johnny from down the street, that grew up as a peace-loving Boy Scout' just did something totally out of character. It quickly and officially was pushed through congress, and classified as a Schedule II substance, with a potential 5 years to life in prison, depending on the amount caught with and perceived intent.

In the beginning, PCP (phencyclidine) was widely embraced by the medical community. In the proper doses, this drug provided effective anesthesia, seemingly without negative effects. However, adverse side effects, including post-operative psychosis, severe anxiety, and dysphoria started getting reported, so the drug was discontinued from human use in 1965.

It was not until the 1960s, during the Haight Ashbury, San Francisco, hippie movement - a culture in search of psychedelic drug use (like LSD) that PCP cropped back up. Its mind-altering effects, and diverse methods of use (snorted, swallowed, smoked, sprayed on) made it popular among that crowd. Smoking PCP, straight or on marijuana, was the most common method of use, according to the DEA (Drug Enforcement Administration).

By 1967, PCP was restricted to "veterinary only" use, rapidly gaining popularity as a tranquilizer. PCP is a white crystalline. Supposedly bitter-tasting powder, which quickly dissolves in water or alcohol, making it easy to 'spray on' pot or other edibles.

Since some people claimed they didn't know they were 'taking it' – because it was being 'sprayed on' their marijuana (or edibles)… and there was not any easy way for the regular users to tell if it what they were buying had been messed with, some unsuspecting people were hurt, and over 80 confirmed deaths in 1978, empowered politicians to push for criminalization.

The most popular street name for it was: 'Angel Dust' – but other names used were: Elephant tranquilizer, Embalming fluid, Killer joints, The PeaCe pill, Rocket fuel, and Supergrass. By 1979, legal manufacturing of PCP in the USA was completely suspended.

I mention this, PCP, only because it was often tied to cannabis in discussions of criminalizing pot in the late 70's. And, as an example of how easy some things can be manipulated and abused by the few irresponsible people that just don't know any better, don't care, and are out to make a quick buck regardless who (or how many) they hurt. Sadly, there were also idiots just looking for their ultimate high (or death).

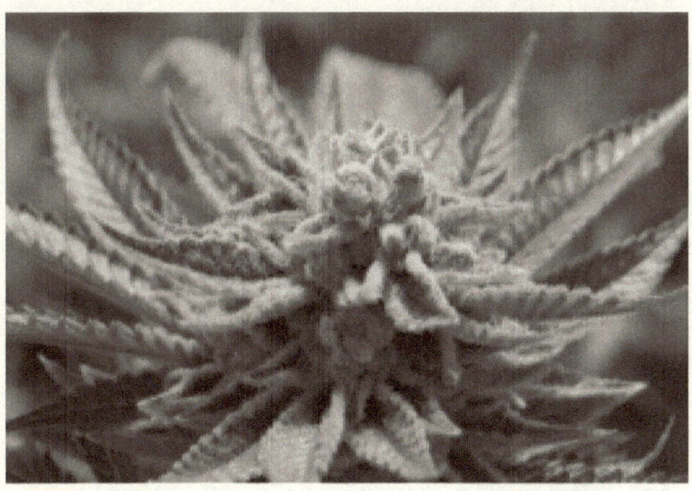

1982, "JUST SAY NO" CAMPAIGN started by Nancy Reagan put the war on drugs back on proverbial steroids of political campaigns, backed by the power of media hype and spin. All those recent actions that included PCP laced marijuana, and LSD abuse, helped pave that way. It was nearly impossible to turn on a TV, or see a newspaper, without hearing all about bad drugs. Mountainous claims, when in fact it was just 'mole hills' of fact, and then only in big cities in this nation (few small towns or rural areas). The rhetoric during the 1980 election campaign was full force.

Most 'hippies' didn't watch tv, or listen to the media, as they were out 'doing their thing' – living in communes, or off the grid, often participating n some Save the Planet, Love the World, NO WAR, NO GOVERMNET or LEAVE ME ALONE campaigns. Some attended college, many lived off the grid. Other than looking or dressing weird, until the Manson Murders and other isolated incidents, most people just viewed them as lazy or strange, because hippies generally did not hurting others.

So prude politicians, that hated 'those lazy anti-war hippies, and all they stood for, as well as the minorities that often used drugs, and the liberal college kids (often living at home still), manipulated by the industry wanting the ban pot, conned the hard working, blue collar working class to demand (or accept) they push through laws to "stop those hippy's" or "Mexicans" from Cheech & Chong's various films.

They labeled 'pot' as a 'gate-way' and 'stepping stone' drug, being convinced 'it' absolutely led to acid, LSD, PCP, heroin… or even those machine gun toting gangsters that were pushing Cocaine, and going to take over this nation, or hurt their kids if those bad people weren't stopped. You know, those you saw in movies like Serpico, Reservoir Dogs, Dirty Harry, McQ, and Scarface. Hollywood ate it up, with their release of block buster, after block buster. People were afraid of those drugged up violent characters (and crimes) in movies like: The Deer Hunter, Midnight Express, Platoon, Apocalypse Now, Less Than Zero, Drugstore Cowboy, A Clockwork Orange, SLC Punk, and even the Die Hard Series.

The government officially classified all forms of cannabis — 'including industrial hemp — as a "Schedule I Drug." That instantly made it illegal to grow, sell, and use in the United States. It was right up there with all the hard drugs that could actually kill people, and completely ruin lives, families, and futures. The 2018 Farm Bill lightened up the federal penalties and controls on Industrial Hemp, but not marijuana or THC... or medical claims.

This one action devastated a whole lot of legal farmers, and agribusinesses. It also forced many American industrial manufacturers' to either re-tool for other raw materials... or import hemp from other countries. Which was still legal, so long as it contained THC levels at, or below, 0.3%. Because it seemed the government thought it was easier to condemn all grown in the USA, but promote cultivation (and trade) in the European Union and Canada. Clearly punishing American farmers.

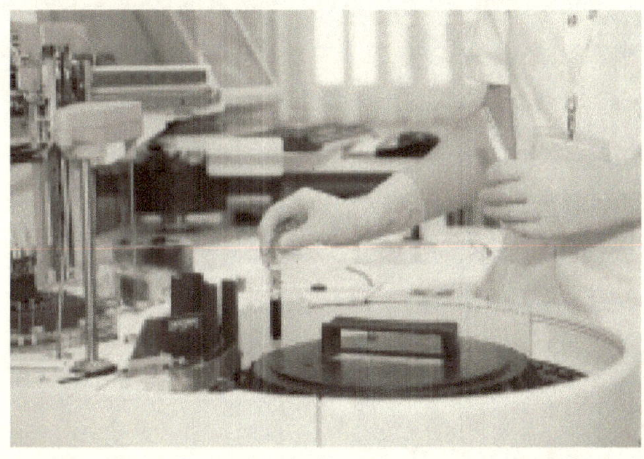

1986, "ANTI-DRUG ABUSE ACT" PASSED (ADAA). This bill established a minimum mandatory prison sentences for certain drug offenses, and then proceeded to pack our nations prisons with non-violent offenders for years. This one action devastated a whole lot of legal farmers, and agribusinesses. It also forced many American industrial manufacturers' to either re-tool for other raw materials... or import hemp from other countries. Which was still legal, for some limited things, so long as it contained THC levels below, 0.3%. The government thought it was easier to condemn all grown in the USA, but promote cultivation (and trade) in the European Union and Canada. Clearly punishing American farmers

2014, Obama Signed A Farm Bill into law, which allowed for the cultivation of industrial hemp (not marijuana, except in those states that have already enacted pro-hemp legislation). This is key, because for the **first time since hemp and marijuana were classified the same in 1970**, a bill in the US government passed into law, acknowledged a slight chemical difference.

However, while some claim 'hemp' was distinctly removed from the definition by Section 7606 of the 2014 Farm bill, which allows and authorizes certain institutions of higher education, and/or the state departments of agriculture, to approve hemp cultivation, under their supervision, regulation, to conduct research and pilot programs... it does NOT 'legalize' hemp products, cannabis products, or CBD Oils for states that haven't otherwise authorized it, unless and until the parties have USDA, FDA, and DEA approval.

There are certainly CBD producers who source their hemp from cultivators that operate under the 2014 Farm Bill, but again, that does NOT legalize or specifically decriminalize sales of it to the general public; at least not UNTIL December 20th, 2018 Farm Bill update was signed into law by President Trump. Another words, you, or I, or Joe/Jill Blow Citizen STILL cannot just up and start an Industrial Hemp grow tomorrow in a state that doesn't otherwise specifically allow it, within their borders and under their rules, just because we feel like it... or someone told us it was legal. **IT IS NOT LEGAL** to grow, possess, or sell in most states.

That Farm Bill allowed the state departments of agriculture and institutions of higher education to cultivate industrial hemp for research purposes. The Bill specifically defines industrial hemp as— "The plant Cannabis sativa L. and any part of such plant, whether growing or not, with a delta-9 tetrahydrocannabinol (THC) concentration of not more than 0.3 percent on a dry weight basis."

2018, 33 States Now Legalizing some to all medical use (22 limited to medical use), but a few have legalized full out private growth and recreational use (11+DC).

With the decriminalization of the Industrial Hemp, and purposeful removal from the Controlled Substance Schedules, and the down grading of marijuana to a lower schedule in the December 20th 2018 Farm Bill President Trump signed into law… it seems that the war on marijuana and CBD Oils might be coming to an end soon. That will necessarily increase the science, studies, stats, and research hopefully answering a variety of questions that have remained unanswered for decades.

However, like most things, it's all subject to change, based on the politicians in power and the cry of the general public claiming to be behind those politicians (law makers). Remember, Carter decriminalized everything in the 70's… three years later it was back on the political chopping block.

Other than the specifically limiting wording on labels and marketing, prohibiting claims, the FDA has zero authority to verify what is 'actually in' any given product that legally falls under DSHEA.

Sarah Campbell, Craft Cannabis Association, in British Columbia, Canada, said "Many small operators envision a day when they can host visitors who can tour their operations and sample the product, as wineries do." October 17th 2018, that is now possible…in Canada.

Watch what HAPPENS WITH the 2018 farm bill, which President Trump signed into Law on December 20th, 2018. Because now the FDA will officially jump into the middle of the regulation of claims and safety… but cleaning the industry up will probably take 3 to 5 years, and everything is frankly **subject to change (when the next president is elected).**

Page Intentionally Left Blank for Your Own Notes:

Page Intentionally Left Blank for Your Own Notes:

WHO PROFITS (Off the 'War On Drugs')

Many times over the years, different donations, political agendas, legislative bills, media campaigns were caught pushing against any legalization to legalize, or even decriminalize anything to do with cannabis, including CBD Oil.

WikiLeaks, in 2016, released a bunch of the DNC (democratic national committee) email transmissions, which showed the party's CONSPIRACY and COLLUSION against 'pot' (marijuana), cannabis products, including CBD. The left might be for it, but many of the politicians they elected to congress sure are not. Notice, the media (and congress) have both been silent about that? Even with the passing of the 2018 Farm Bill, on the 20th of December 2018... just days before Christmas. Crickets.

Well, the sad reality is that there are multiple industries that love the 'war on drugs,' and have been profiting off exactly that for many years. Some of these are:

A. ILLEGAL DRUG SUPPLIERS/MANUFACTURERS – so long as the government helps keep the supply low, and the addicts and ignorant keep the demand up, the price will always be as high as possible, which in turn promotes the side effect of crime… so the addicts can pay for their habit.

It seems the 'black market' flourishes in many parts of the world. America is not immune, with some cities even 'giving away' syringes, claiming they are reducing the spread of AIDS and other diseases. Yet Diabetics that can't afford insurance don't get much free or low cost help.

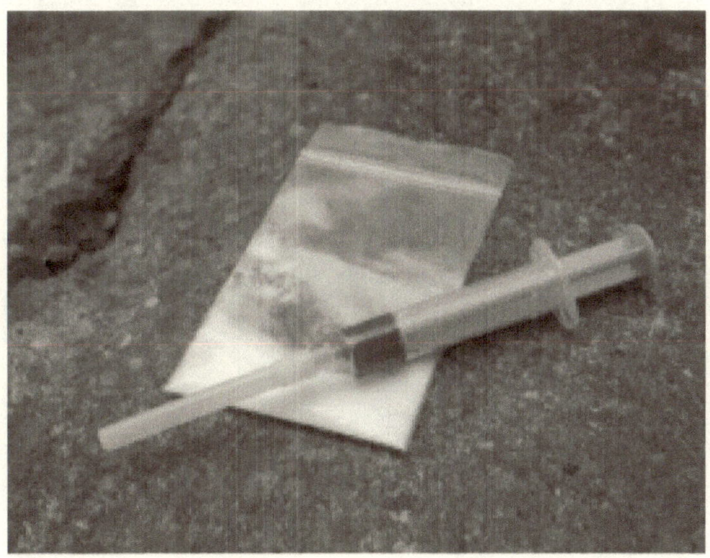

B. **HERBAL SUPPLEMENTS** (Promoting Synthetic Highs) – and masking pain and other symptoms. There are a whole bunch of herbal companies, and holistic supplement suppliers, that ignore science, abuse and twist the reality of science, and sell the illusion of 'getting better' by merely covering up symptoms, not healing anything. They target those people that want to 'be legal' and 'above the law,' yet want to 'kill their pain' – escape their reality – and hope to treat some ailment without the expense of a real doctor, surgery, or prescription drugs.

They want to self-medicate, and have more control for less cost (in their mind), to reduce or eliminate symptoms… without using 'street drugs' or alcohol.

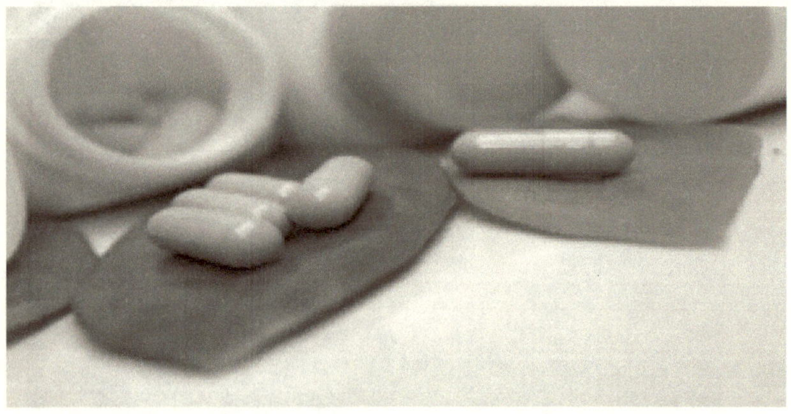

C. DRUG TESTING INDUSTRY – who would have thought? But the reality is that either the government or employer requires the drug tests… and sometimes the hospital for treatment purposes, or the police for their self- protection (or criminal charges). Sadly, it is often the 'tax-payers' that pays for the testing, regardless of the results.

If the person passes, that cost was deemed a waste. If the person fails, they usually do not get any help… they just get turned down from whatever they were applying for, denied coverage, or fired. All of those results create an interesting conundrum, and pretty much a 'damned if you do vs damned if you don't' type scenario, which seldom exists with alcohol, or any other individualized recreational activity. It is one thing if someone is (or might likely be) hurt because of an intoxicated persons actions. It is quite another what some adult does in the confines of their own home, without endangering anyone else.

However, there has been a big push, the last few years, for testing of every person living off the taxpayers, particularly welfare recipients. In one example, published in the NY Times, 17 April 2012, Ms. Lizette Alvarez claimed "Florida State spent $118,140 drug testing welfare applicants, which was $45,780 more than they would have spent if they would have just given the welfare to those same 108 applicants that tested positive for drugs."

Clearly, that reporter was better at creative writing than mathematics, as the claim was what is called 'magic math.' It ignorantly supported their agenda, with short sighted and less than honest information. They failed to take into account a whole lot of other necessary factors… but especially the actual monthly allotment those 108 failed applicants would have otherwise been getting.

The NYT math works out to: ($118,140+$45,780)/108=$1517.77 per failed household/applicant. We all know that is not a lifetime or annualized, or even quarterly figure… therefore multiply it by 12 months, by number of applicants, equals an annualized savings of $1,967,029.92 in cash welfare benefits (not including interest, or the other cost factors that might have otherwise been occurred) by Florida State.

Now, the numbers also do not account for what happens to the children (or how many of those 108 applicants failing the drug tests, or the 50 that did not take the test because they knew they would fail, had children). Or how those children were otherwise cared for.

Or if there was an increase in crime by those failed cases, or any other taxpayer funded costs (such as hospital, jail, police, mental health, court system, foster care, etc.).

Now, in Ms. Alvarez's defense, it sounded like she just bought into the hyperbole (and malformed numbers) of Derek Newton, communications director for the ACLU of Florida, whom she quoted. Shame on them both for promoting obviously flawed and disingenuous short-sighted information!

D. ALCOHOL (AND BEER) INDUSTRY – "Pot is safer than alcohol" and "No one has ever died from a marijuana overdose" are two factors the alcohol industry tries to avoid, and market around.

Many of the alcohol distributors helps fund, and lobby for, the criminalization of marijuana. They love less competition, especially when the strong arm of the taxpayer funded government is limiting or eliminating their competition. Over a five-year period, just **1.8 percent of fatal crashes involved drivers who tested positive only for cannabis.**

However, in Nevada, records indicate that the alcohol industry is among the biggest donors to PRO-legalization, according to the Center for Public Integrity. **However**, interestingly, most of the Nevada initiative would hand alcohol distributors the SOLE RIGHT to sell cannabis for the first 18 months.

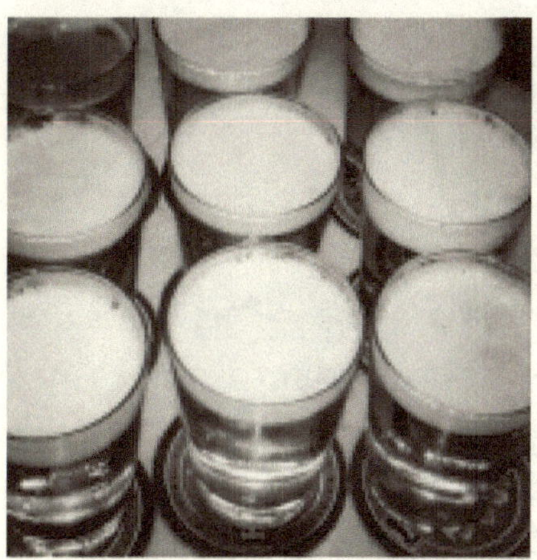

E. **PRIVATE PRISON INDUSTRY** – including the prison guard/staff unions, but it is more than just 'job security.' CCA (Corrections Corp. of America) and Cornell Group are the largest private prison companies. They seem to play both ends against the middle, lobbying and donating big bucks to secure and grow their position. They also supply drug-sniffing dogs, and other tools, to help capture those nasty drug abusers. (sorry, sarcastic font missing) It is estimated that over 50% of the current prison population is a direct result of the 'war on drugs.' Consider their own words:

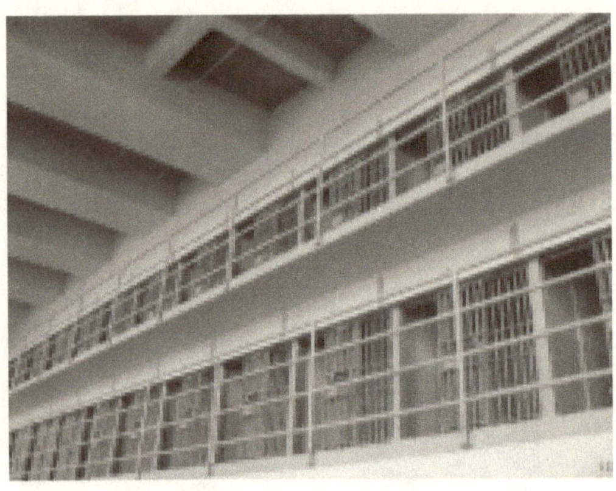

"The demand for our facilities and services could be adversely affected by the relaxation of enforcement efforts, leniency in conviction or parole standards and sentencing practices or through the decriminalization of certain activities that are currently proscribed by our criminal laws. For instance, any changes with respect to drugs and controlled substances or illegal immigration could affect the number of persons arrested, convicted, and sentenced, thereby potentially reducing demand for correctional facilities to house them.

Legislation has been proposed in numerous jurisdictions that could lower minimum sentences for some non-violent crimes and make more inmates eligible for early release based on good behavior.

Also, sentencing alternatives under consideration could put some offenders on probation with electronic monitoring who would otherwise be incarcerated. Similarly, reductions in crime rates or resources dedicated to prevent and enforce crime could lead to reductions in arrests, convictions and sentences requiring incarceration at correctional facilities." ~ CORRECTIONS CORPORATION OF AMERICA 2010 ANNUAL REPORT

Consider, for a moment, the state AND federal prison population increased 722% between 1970 and 2009! From just 196,429 inmates in 1970, to 1,613,740 on the first day of 2009. Worse, as of 2018, the privatized prisons account for only 8% of the inmates, but still rake in billions each year.

F. **ADDICTION RECOVERY INDUSTRY** - this does not mean there are not voluntary clients. It's that those 'in power' (of that industry) want government to officially declare drug use a disease; which, then, forces anyone who is deemed to have the disease to receive very specific treatment, from very specific doctors, and then have a third party pay the bill.

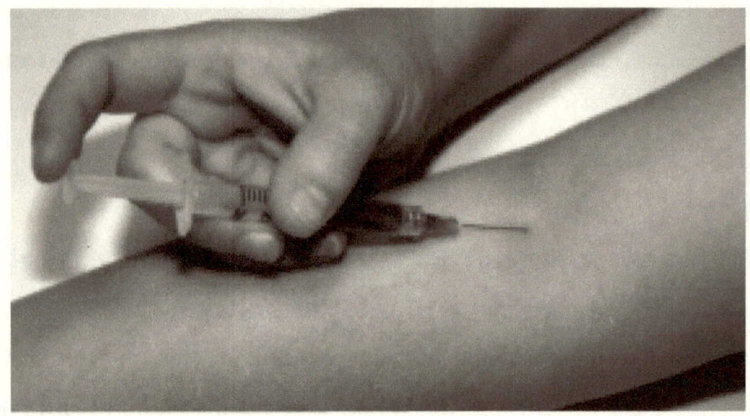

G. JUDICIAL SYSTEM - The sad part is that the police (unions), judges, court system, jails, public prison system… and assorted support staff… all add up to a whole lot of good paying jobs. Sadly, the employment numbers, all funded by the taxpayers, are justified by the NUMBER OF PRISONERS… and the system.

Our nation's judicial system not only helps justify a pile of different jobs, and need for larger jails, courts, after release support systems, etc. but also has a direct impact on starting a cycle of watching, and recidivism, because over 83% are statistically likely to re-offend within the first five years, according to the Department of Justice 2018 study entitled "2018 Update on Prisoner Recidivism: A 9-Year Follow-up Period (2005-2014) ".

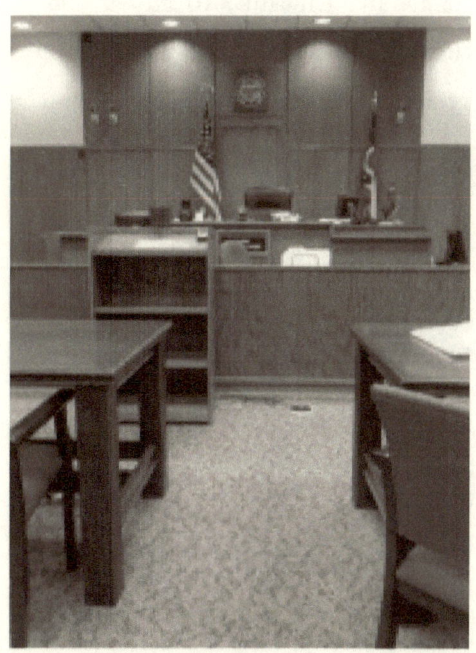

The results of that 30 state study proves the cycle is perpetuating what the war on drugs helped start. It's also important to understand that, because many of those 'convicted' of Schedule 1 substances are now lifetime 'felons' with fewer civil rights, there is a higher likelihood of escalating to bigger crimes, just for them to hope to 'stay out' of prison, or just survive and build a family in the future.

Arresting non-violent offenders, that have not hurt anyone... aren't victimizing others... aren't pushing 'hard' drugs known to ruin or endanger lives, (like meth, PCP, rape drugs, or designer drugs) cost society in more ways than one. Just like the alcohol prohibition's failure, by now it should be abundantly clear that minimum mandatory sentences are not working, especially for things like cannabis. To further complicate things, these non-violent 'criminals' are stuck in the taxpayer funded system, longer than many burglars, robbers, rapists, and even murders. How's that for real justice?

H. **BIG PHARMA** - Purdue Pharma (OxyContin) and Abbott Laboratories (Vicodin) are among the largest contributors to the Anti-Drug Coalition of America, according to reports. Clearly, with the Veteran's Affairs ceasing nearly all of their regular monthly prescriptions mailed out to veterans with chronic pain management issues hurt big pharma, costing them hundreds of millions of dollars, in one decision.

According to Alfonso Serrano, of The Guardian, "Opiate overdoses dropped by nearly 25% in states that have legalized medical marijuana, compared to states that prohibited sales, according to a 2014 study from the Journal of the American Medical Association. The study implies that people could be using medical marijuana to treat their pain, rather than opioid painkillers, or they are taking lower doses. Research published this year, by the University of Georgia, shows **Medicare prescriptions for drugs used to treat chronic pain and anxiety dropped significantly in states that have legalized medical marijuana.** Medicare saved roughly $165m in 2013 according to the study, which estimated that expenditures for Medicare Part D, the portion of the government-funded health insurance program that subsidizes prescription drug costs, **would drop by over $470m annually if medical marijuana were legalized nationally."**

OyxContin, Hydrocodone, and Vicodin, which were all 100% FDA approved, cost our nation thousands of lives each year, from people merely wanting to eliminate, reduce, or control chronic pain. According to the CDC, over 200,000 deaths occurred from opioid abuse, over doses, between 1999 and 2016. Prescription Drugs are directly related to more than 300% more deaths than all illegal drugs. In just 2017, more than 72,000 Americans died from drug overdoses (note: the sharpest increase occurred among deaths related to fentanyl and fentanyl analogs (synthetic opioids) with nearly 30,000 overdose deaths).

To date, with over 4,000 years of written history, there has not been one person anywhere in the world has died from a cannabis overdose, or marijuana abuse.

Page Intentionally Left Blank for Your Own Notes:

Celebrities – Athletes, Actors, Politicians

These people have either publicly said or done something that put them in the media for cannabis use…

Ross Rebagliati, Gold Medal snow boarder on the world stage, after his fiasco in 1998, which led to a full on ban of marijuana in 1999 for all Olympic athletes. However, the rules changed again, in 2013, lightening up to allow up to 150ng/ml of THC in the blood stream. Accepting that some Olympians may consume marijuana products <u>in the off season for valid medical reasons</u>, but still banning use during active competition, according to the WADA (World Anti-Doping Agency).

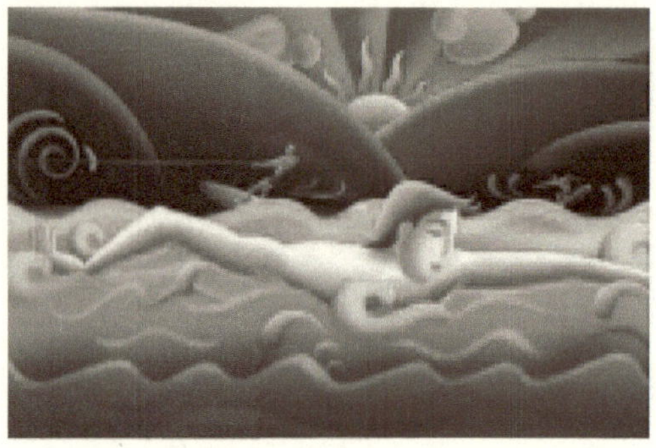

Michael Phelps, the human fish, the man with 28 Olympic medals, 23 Gold, more than any other person alive. He is also the holder of multiple world records, and unintentionally helped bring to light that weed is not just for 'stoners' or 'losers,' but potentially even star athletes that require optimum breathing. Phelps won eight medals at the 2004 Athens Olympics, eight in Beijing in 2008, six in London in 2012 and six more in Rio. He tested clean during each of the Olympic Games.

The world's fastest man, Usain Bolt, admitted to smoking marijuana when he was young, growing up in Jamaica.

But 2012 US Judoka Nicholas Delpopolo was expelled from competition after he tested positive for cannabis (THC). He said he did not know there was pot inside a brownie he ate at a celebration party with friends, and called it "the worst thing I have ever done in my life."

Athletes – both Olympians and Professionals, many celebrities – actors, actresses, and musicians, the parents of severely ill children, and people battling cancer, epilepsy, chronic pain, eating or sleep disorders, and assorted other issues use cannabis products to 'self-medicate.' People have been speaking out publicly about their personal experience with cannabis for about 30 years now.

This is just a list of a few that have publicly spoke out. Actor Robert Mitchum was not the first celebrity to 'be caught' using marijuana, just one the federal government attempted to make an example of in 1948 when he was arrested during a private party. Hugh Hefner, Bob Marley, Drake, Miley Cyrus, Jimi Hendrix, Jerry Garcia, Cheech & Chong, Kirsten Dunst, Brad Pitt, Woody Harrelson, The Beatles, Lil Wayne, Seth Rogen, Cameron Diaz, Matthew McConaughey, Steve Jobs, Whoopi Goldberg, Kyuss, Cypress Hill, Willie Nelson, Ricky Williams, Ronda Rousey, Ben and Jerry, Kevin Smith (Silent Bob), Roseanne Barr, Nate Diaz, Nick Diaz, Kareen Abdul-Jabbar, Rob Van Dam, Anna Faris, Sarah Silverman, and tens of thousands more, still 'in the closet'… quietly using behind the scenes.

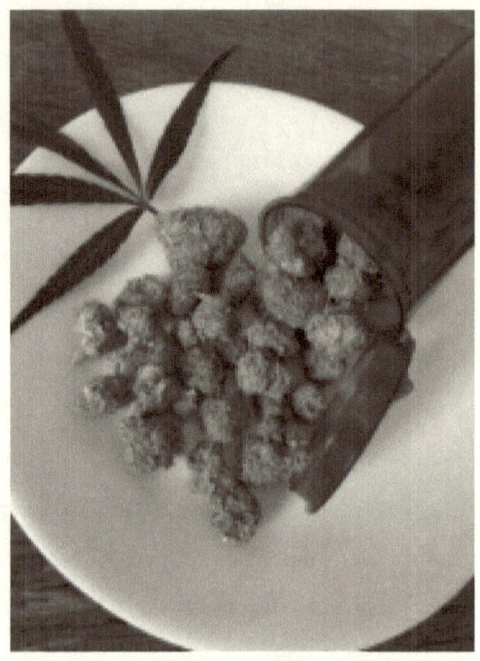

Even politicians, from both sides of the aisle, George Washington, Benjamin Franklin, Thomas Jefferson, James Madison, Bill "but I didn't inhale" Clinton, George W. Bush, and Obama; Sarah Palin, Jeb Bush, Arnold Schwarzenegger, John Edwards, Newt Gingrich, John Kerry, Jesse Ventura, Al Gore, Howard Dean, Michael Bloomberg, Andrew Cuomo, Gary Johnson, Joseph P. Kennedy II, George Pataki, Clarence Thomas, have all admitted to smoking marijuana, at least once. The reality is the true list would include thousands of politicians from around the world over just the last couple hundred years. It would include persons in political power, past and present, and in the media. Likely rivaling the number of people that still drank alcohol more than once or twice a year during the prohibition.

This page is for your Notes:

CONCLUSION

Science is interesting. The numbers might be skewed in their reading, or reporting, but ultimately they generally do not lie, if you know which to look for, and what questions to ask.

Health and healing are vital to quality of life and longevity, so we decided to dig deeper on the topics of 'health' and 'alternative health' over the last twenty years. .

The potential benefits of quality vitamins, minerals, amino acids, enzymes, and modern medicine (such as necessary vaccines, antibiotics, and key drugs) is exactly why most of us are alive today. We know this, cherish that fact.

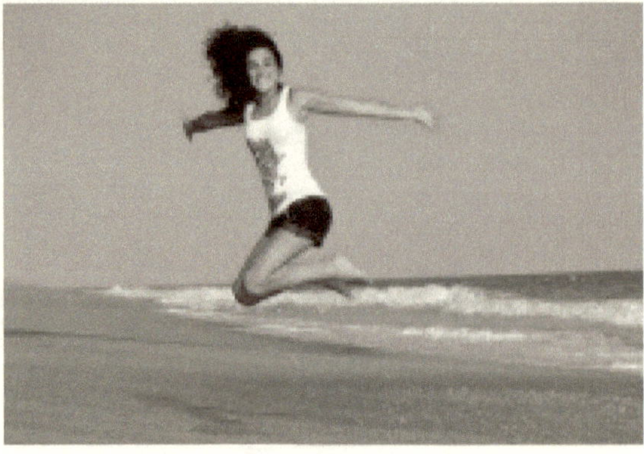

Learning, inventions, and improvements of knowledge, application, and consistency in process is vital to the future of this world. To our family, friends, and maybe even clients science is absolutely important.

We spent a lot of time wading through the research, studies, and claims… to determine just how much is real, what it *might* actually do, how it actually does, and what is hype (smoke and mirrors, marketing magic, problems with the claims, and outright lies there might be).

ACKNOWLEDGEMENTS

Mrs. Carly Mercer, my other half, wife, and partner, A Special Thanks for both the patience while I'm researching and writing stuff… and for all the time spent editing, helping catch any grammar and spelling errors (which were copious). Her suggestions and questions really helped, and she really helped improve the quality of the information contained within. She takes great care of me and keeps me healthier, while making me happier. I am better because of her

With a special thanks to my kids, **Tevyn**, **Tyler** and my daughter-in-law, **Erikka**, **Talya**, and **Kristopher**; my sisters and their families, and my parents, all of which helped give me the motivation to keep putting one foot in front of the other, and doing the best I can to and accomplish positive things in my life… and to help others when possible.

Amy Davis, my Cousin, who went through word by word, finding a few type-os, and asking a bunch of questions that were as clearly answered in the last draft.

Dr. David F. Davenport, DVM, MS, MS, CNS for input on what cannabis studies show it can (and actually can't) really do to arthritis, and the concerns messing the immune system response.

Russ Leamons, for tossing out some additional ideas and concepts to research and either prove or disprove, with science.

Ron & Michelle Coffman, friends for decades, from junior high school, that help edit and make suggestions… and banter ideas and information.

Frank McAlister, for his time in looking through the information and helping catch any mistakes, errors, and type-o's; and the input on different types of Epilepsy. Because of Frank, I was able to actually have time with my children living on the west coast more often than most estranged father's living in the same town. For that I'm forever grateful! He held down the office, and fort, while I was on the road between trade shows, exhibits, events, calling on clients, and spending time with my kids as much as I could for over a decade, despite living over 3,000 miles away from them.

Dr. James Bailey, PhD Nutritionist and Clinical Instructor, retired for some of the insight on how some things function and work within the body, and how to evaluate the research through abstracts, third party studies, and peer reviewed journal articles.

Photos/images – used under license from **Digital Juice** (incredible quality images, videos, and sounds for commercial use… at a reasonable cost), or CC (Creative Commons) License from **Pixabay.com** (over 1.5 Million royalty free stock images), or one of the other resources we've invested in over the years.

LEGALESE

All rights reserved. No part of this publication, or the information in it, may be quoted from or reproduced in any for, by any means, such as printing, scanning, photocopying, tangibly or digitally, for any reasons, **without prior written permission of the copyright holder.**

Neither the Author, nor the Publisher or any Reseller, in no way encourages illegal activity and would like to remind its readers that marijuana usage, as well as the consumable products created from cannabis, continues to be an offense under Federal Law, regardless of state marijuana laws.

Efforts have been made to help ensure that the information contained in this book are accurate, complete, explained well, and unbiased.

The author and the publisher do not make any warranty of the information, text, or graphics contained herein due to the rapidly changing nature of science, research, laws, and policies, and variables in other countries, known and unknown. The graphics used are general, generic, to help break up the monotony of the sometimes technical and scientific text. Neither the Author or Publisher hold the copyrights for the graphics, they are used under license; either a purchase, membership subscription, or creative commons.

The Author and publisher do not hold any responsibility for errors, omissions, or contrary interpretations of anything contained herein.

This book is presented strictly for informational and educational purposes, and the **Author suggests the reader should consult their healthcare provider** for any medical concerns, or treatment; and/or their lawyer, if there are any actual legal concerns.

Nothing contained in this book has been evaluated or approved by the FDA, and nothing herein is intended to offer medical or legal advice, nor any cure, treatment, or preventive measures for any disease or health issue. Consult a licensed professional that can help deal with your specific unique case and situation.

REFERENCES

http://www.cureyourowncancer.org/dennis-hills-story-beating-prostate-cancer-

http://www.cureyourowncancer.org/the-kelly-hauf-story-how-she-beat-brain-

http://www.thecannabist.co/2016/08/11/dea-reschedule-marijuana-rules-federal-register/60777/

http://www.thecannabist.co/2016/08/11/dea-reschedule-marijuana-rules-federal-register/60777/

https://herb.co/marijuana/news/naming-mile-high-stadium

https://news.medicalmarijuanainc.com/the-road-to-prohibition-why-did-america-make-marijuana-illegal-in-the-first-place/

https://www.cdc.gov/mmwr/volumes/67/wr/mm6720a5.htm?s_cid=mm6720a5_x

DHHS Letter to Chuck Rosenberg

https://www.deadiversion.usdoj.gov/schedules/marijuana/Acting_Administrator_Rosenberg_Response_to_Request_Marijuana_Rescheduling.pdf#search=cbd

https://www.denverpost.com/2016/08/28/what-is-marijuana-patent-6630507/

https://www.leafscience.com/2014/07/25/u-s-government-patent-marijuana/

https://www.naturalproductsinsider.com/videos/2018/01/gw-pharmaceuticals.aspx

https://www.spandidos-publications.com/10.3892/or.2015.3746

https://www.youtube.com/watch?time_continue=10&v=dSI-U4U62E

[Therapeutical use of the cannabinoids in psychiatry]. Rev Bras Psiquiatr 32 (Suppl 1): S56-66, 2010. Crippa JA, Zuardi AW, Hallak JE: [PUBMED Abstract]

A combined preclinical therapy of cannabinoids and temozolomide against glioma. Mol Cancer Ther 10 (1): 90-103, 2011. Torres S, Lorente M, Rodríguez-Fornés F, et al.: [PUBMED Abstract]

Activation of cannabinoid CB1 and CB2 receptors suppresses neuropathic nociception evoked by the chemotherapeutic agent vincristine in rats. Br J Pharmacol 152 (5): 765-77, 2007. Rahn EJ, Makriyannis A, Hohmann AG: [PUBMED Abstract]

Addiction. 1996 Nov;91(11):1585-614.
Cannabis: pharmacology and toxicology in animals and humans. Adams IB, Martin BR.
https://www.ncbi.nlm.nih.gov/pubmed/8972919

An analgesia circuit activated by cannabinoids. Nature 395 (6700): 381-3, 1998. Meng ID, Manning BH, Martin WJ, et al.:
[PUBMED Abstract]

Antianxiety effect of cannabidiol in the elevated plus-maze. Psychopharmacology (Berl) 100 (4): 558-9, 1990. Guimarães FS, Chiaretti TM, Graeff FG, et al.:
[PUBMED Abstract]

Antidepressant and Anxiolytic like effect of Cannabidiol
Antidepressant-Like and Anxiolytic-Like Effects of Cannabidiol- A Chemical Compound of Cannabis sativa.pdf

Antidepressant-like and anxiolytic-like effects of cannabidiol: a chemical compound of Cannabis sativa. CNS Neurol Disord Drug Targets. 2014;13(6):953-60. de Mello Schier AR, de Oliveira Ribeiro NP, Coutinho DS, Machado S, Arias-Carrión O, Crippa JA, Zuardi AW, Nardi AE, Silva AC
https://www.ncbi.nlm.nih.gov/pubmed/24923339

Antiemetic effect of delta-9-tetrahydrocannabinol in patients receiving cancer chemotherapy. N Engl J Med 293 (16): 795-7, 1975. [PUBMED Abstract] Sallan SE, Zinberg NE, Frei E 3rd:

http://www.ncbi.nlm.nih.gov/entrez/query.fcgi?cmd=Retrieve&db=Pub
Med&list_uids=1099449&dopt=Abstract

Anti-tumoral action of cannabinoids on hepatocellular carcinoma: role
of AMPK-dependent activation of autophagy. Cell Death Differ 18 (7):
1099-111, 2011. Vara D, Salazar M, Olea-Herrero N, et al.:
[PUBMED Abstract]

As of September 20th, 2018 – directly from the VA Website:
https://www.publichealth.va.gov/marijuana.asp

Bey, T., & Patel, A. (2007).
Phencyclidine Intoxication and Adverse Effects: A Clinical and
Pharmacological Review of an Illicit Drug. The California Journal of
Emergency Medicine, 8(1), 9–14.

Braz J Med Biol Res. 2006 Apr;39(4):421-9. Epub 2006 Apr 3.
https://www.ncbi.nlm.nih.gov/pmc/articles/PMC2859735/

Brenner, S, Corden, T.E., Dribben, W.H., Windle, M.L., & Tucker, J.R.
(2014). PCP Toxicity
https://www.google.co.uk/patents/US6630507

California Narcotic Officers' Association (n.d.). THE PCP STORY.
Retrieved September 9, 2015, from
https://www.cnoa.org/documents/NPCP.pdf

Can Marijuana Kill Your Dog? By Russ Belville

https://www.alternet.org/drugs/can-marijuana-kill-your-dog

Cannabidiol enhances the inhibitory effects of delta9-tetrahydrocannabinol on human glioblastoma cell proliferation and survival. Mol Cancer Ther 9 (1): 180-9, 2010. Marcu JP, Christian RT, Lau D, et al.:
[PUBMED Abstract]

Cannabidiol induces programmed cell death in breast cancer cells by coordinating the cross-talk between apoptosis and autophagy. Mol Cancer Ther 10 (7): 1161-72, 2011 Shrivastava A, Kuzontkoski PM, Groopman JE, et al.:
[PUBMED Abstract]

Cannabidiol inhibits human glioma cell migration through a cannabinoid receptor-independent mechanism. Br J Pharmacol 144 (8): 1032-6, 2005. Vaccani A, Massi P, Colombo A, et al.:
[PUBMED Abstract]

Cannabidiol inhibits lung cancer cell invasion and metastasis via intercellular adhesion molecule-1. FASEB J 26 (4): 1535-48, 2012. Ramer R, Bublitz K, Freimuth N, et al.:
[PUBMED Abstract]

Cannabidiol inhibits paclitaxel-induced neuropathic pain through 5-HT(1A) receptors without diminishing nervous system function or chemotherapy efficacy. Br J Pharmacol 171 (3): 636-45, 2014. Ward SJ, McAllister SD, Kawamura R, et al.:

[PUBMED Abstract]

Cannabinoid receptors and their endogenous agonists. Annu Rev
Pharmacol Toxicol 38: 179-200, 1998. [PUBMED Abstract] Felder CC,
Glass M:
http://www.ncbi.nlm.nih.gov/entrez/query.fcgi?cmd=Retrieve&db=Pub
Med&list_uids=9597153&dopt=Abstract

Cannabinoid receptors in brain: pharmacogenetics, neuropharmacology,
neurotoxicology, and potential therapeutic applications. Onaivi ES.
Int Rev Neurobiol. 2009;88:335-69. doi: 10.1016/S0074-
7742(09)88012-4.
https://www.ncbi.nlm.nih.gov/pubmed/19897083

Cannabinoid receptors, CB1 and CB2, as novel targets for inhibition of
non-small cell lung cancer growth and metastasis. Cancer Prev Res
(Phila) 4 (1): 65-75, 2011. Preet A, Qamri Z, Nasser MW, et al.:
[PUBMED Abstract]

Cannabinoid type-1 receptor reduces pain and neurotoxicity produced by
chemotherapy. J Neurosci 32 (20): 7091-101, 2012. Khasabova IA,
Khasabov S, Paz J, et al.:
[PUBMED Abstract]

Cannabinoids and cancer: potential for colorectal cancer therapy.
Biochem Soc Trans 33 (Pt 4): 712-4, 2005. Patsos HA, Hicks DJ,
Greenhough A, et al.:
[PUBMED Abstract]

Cannabinoids and cancer: pros and cons of an antitumour strategy. Br J
Pharmacol 148 (2): 123-35, 2006. Bifulco M, Laezza C, Pisanti S, et al.:
[PUBMED Abstract]

Cannabinoids for cancer treatment: progress and promise. Cancer Res 68
(2): 339-42, 2008. Sarfaraz S, Adhami VM, Syed DN, et al.:
[PUBMED Abstract]

Cannabinoids inhibit the vascular endothelial growth factor pathway in
gliomas. Cancer Res 64 (16): 5617-23, 2004. Blázquez C, González-
Feria L, Alvarez L, et al.:
[PUBMED Abstract]

Cannabinoids reduce ErbB2-driven breast cancer progression through
Akt inhibition. Mol Cancer 9: 196, 2010. Caffarel MM, Andradas C,
Mira E, et al.:
[PUBMED Abstract]

Cannabinoids reduce hyperalgesia and inflammation via interaction with
peripheral CB1 receptors. Pain 75 (1): 111-9, 1998. Richardson JD, Kilo
S, Hargreaves KM:
[PUBMED Abstract]

Cannabinoids. J Pain Symptom Manage 46 (1): 142-9, 2013. Howard P,
Twycross R, Shuster J, et al.: [PUBMED Abstract]
http://www.ncbi.nlm.nih.gov/entrez/query.fcgi?cmd=Retrieve&db=Pub
Med&list_uids=23707385&dopt=Abstract

Cannabinoids: potential anticancer agents. Nat Rev Cancer 3 (10): 745-55, 2003. Guzmán M:
[PUBMED Abstract]

Cannabidiol, a Cannabis sativa constituent, as an antipsychotic drug. Zuardi AW1, Crippa JA, Hallak JE, Moreira FA, Guimarães FS.
https://www.ncbi.nlm.nih.gov/pubmed/16612464

Cannabis and Cannabinoids: Pharmacology, Toxicology, and Therapeutic Potential. Binghamton, NY: The Haworth Press, 2002. Grotenhermen F, Russo E, eds.:
https://www.researchgate.net/publication/237399814_Cannabis_and_Cannabinoids_Pharmacology_Toxicology_and_Therapeutic_Potential

Cannabis and Insurance Last Updated 2/16/18
https://www.naic.org/cipr_topics/topic_cannabis_and_insurance.htm

Cannabis: A History. New York, NY: St Martin's Press, 2003. Booth M:
https://www.amazon.com/Cannabis-History-Martin-Booth-ebook/dp/B00Y7S51TQ

Cannabis: pharmacology and toxicology in animals and humans. Addiction 91 (11): 1585-614, 1996. Adams IB, Martin BR:
[PUBMED Abstract]

Cannabis-derived substances in cancer therapy--an emerging anti-inflammatory role for the cannabinoids. Curr Clin Pharmacol 5 (4): 281-

7, 2010. Liu WM, Fowler DW, Dalgleish AG:
[PUBMED Abstract]

CB1 and CB2 receptor agonists promote analgesia through synergy in a
murine model of tumor pain. Behav Pharmacol 22 (5-6): 607-16, 2011.
Khasabova IA, Gielissen J, Chandiramani A, et al.:
[PUBMED Abstract]

CB2 cannabinoid receptor activation produces antinociception by
stimulating peripheral release of endogenous opioids. Proc Natl Acad
Sci U S A 102 (8): 3093-8, 2005. Ibrahim MM, Porreca F, Lai J, et al.:
[PUBMED Abstract]

CBD oil is illegal in Alabama
https://www.timesdaily.com/news/crime/cbd-oil-is-illegal-in-
alabama/article_e637229a-101e-59c2-a499-1721c5e06902.html

CBD Outrage: 36 Hours in Jail for CBD Oil Sold at Grocery Store
https://www.leafly.com/news/politics/cbd-outrage-36-hours-in-jail-for-
cbd-oil-sold-at-grocery-store

Chemistry, Metabolism, and Toxicology of Cannabis: Clinical
Implications Priyamvada Sharma, PhD,corresponding author1 Pratima
Murthy,1 and M.M. Srinivas Bharath2
https://www.ncbi.nlm.nih.gov/pmc/articles/PMC3570572/

Chemopreventive effect of the non-psychotropic phytocannabinoid
cannabidiol on experimental colon cancer. J Mol Med (Berl) 90 (8):

925-34, 2012. Aviello G, Romano B, Borrelli F, et al.:
[PUBMED Abstract]

Colorado marijuana sales since January 2014 reach $5 billion
https://www.summitdaily.com/news/marijuana/colorado-marijuana-sales-since-january-2014-reach-5-billion/

Colorado pot sales hit a record $1.5 billion in 2017, and border towns saw a green rush from neighbors
https://www.denverpost.com/2018/02/10/colorado-pot-sales-2017-border-towns/

Critical appraisal of the potential use of cannabinoids in cancer management. Cancer Manag Res 5: 301-13, 2013. Cridge BJ, Rosengren RJ:
[PUBMED Abstract]

Crosstalk between chemokine receptor CXCR4 and cannabinoid receptor CB2 in modulating breast cancer growth and invasion. PLoS One 6 (9): e23901, 2011. Nasser MW, Qamri Z, Deol YS, et al.:
[PUBMED Abstract]

Curr Pharm Des. 2014;20(13):2194-204.
Cannabinoids and schizophrenia: therapeutic prospects. Robson PJ, Guy GW, Di Marzo V1.
https://www.ncbi.nlm.nih.gov/pubmed/23829368

DEA Internal Directive Regarding the Presence of Cannabinoids in

Products and Materials Made from the Cannabis Plant (May 22, 2018)
https://www.deadiversion.usdoj.gov/schedules/marijuana/dea_internal_d
irective_cannabinoids_05222018.html

DEA: Feds won't arrest CBD oil users, neither should Indiana
https://www.wthr.com/article/dea-feds-wont-arrest-cbd-oil-users-
neither-should-indiana

Dealing with Medical Marijuana 07/22/16
https://medicaljustice.com/dealing-medical-marijuana/

Delta(9)-tetrahydrocannabinol and synthetic cannabinoids prevent
emesis produced by the cannabinoid CB(1) receptor antagonist/inverse
agonist SR 141716A. Neuropsychopharmacology 24 (2): 198-203, 2001.
Darmani NA:
[PUBMED Abstract]

Delta-9-tetrahydrocannabinol differentially suppresses cisplatin-induced
emesis and indices of motor function via cannabinoid CB(1) receptors in
the least shrew. Pharmacol Biochem Behav 69 (1-2): 239-49, 2001 May-
Jun. Darmani NA:
[PUBMED Abstract]

Delta-9-tetrahydrocannabinol enhances breast cancer growth and
metastasis by suppression of the antitumor immune response. J Immunol
174 (6): 3281-9, 2005. McKallip RJ, Nagarkatti M, Nagarkatti PS:
[PUBMED Abstract]

Delta-9-tetrahydrocannabinol inhibits antitumor immunity by a CB2 receptor-mediated, cytokine-dependent pathway. J Immunol 165 (1): 373-80, 2000. Zhu LX, Sharma S, Stolina M, et al.:
[PUBMED Abstract]

Delta9-Tetrahydrocannabinol inhibits epithelial growth factor-induced lung cancer cell migration in vitro as well as its growth and metastasis in vivo. Oncogene 27 (3): 339-46, 2008. Preet A, Ganju RK, Groopman JE:
[PUBMED Abstract]

Department of Health & Human Services (2011). National Survey on Drug Use and Health Summary: Report of Findings. DHHS.
http://archive.samhsa.gov/data/NSDUH/2k11Results/NSDUHresults2011.htm

Department of Health & Human Services (The DAWN Report: Club Drugs, 2002 Update. July 2004.
http://dawninfo.samhsa.gov/old_dawn/pubs_94_02/shortreports/files/DAWN_tdr_club_drugs02.pdf

Determination and characterization of a cannabinoid receptor in rat brain. Mol Pharmacol 34 (5): 605-13, 1988. [PUBMED Abstract] Devane WA, Dysarz FA 3rd, Johnson MR, et al.
http://www.ncbi.nlm.nih.gov/entrez/query.fcgi?cmd=Retrieve&db=PubMed&list_uids=2848184&dopt=Abstract

DHHS Letter to Chuck Rosenberg

Acting Administrator Rosenberg Response to request for Marijuana...
https://www.deadiversion.usdoj.gov/schedules/marijuana/Incoming_Lett
er_Department%20_HHS.pdf#search=cbd

Distinct effects of {delta}9-tetrahydrocannabinol and cannabidiol on
neural activation during emotional processing. Arch Gen Psychiatry.
2009 Jan;66(1):95-105. doi: 10.1001/archgenpsychiatry.2008.519.
Fusar-Poli P1, Crippa JA, Bhattacharyya S, Borgwardt SJ, Allen P,
Martin-Santos R, Seal M, Surguladze SA, O'Carrol C, Atakan Z, Zuardi
AW, McGuire PK.
https://www.ncbi.nlm.nih.gov/pubmed/19124693

Dronabinol as a treatment for anorexia associated with weight loss in
patients with AIDS. J Pain Symptom Manage 10 (2): 89-97, 1995.
[PUBMED Abstract] Beal JE, Olson R, Laubenstein L, et al.
http://www.ncbi.nlm.nih.gov/entrez/query.fcgi?cmd=Retrieve&db=Pub
Med&list_uids=7730690&dopt=Abstract

Dronabinol effects on weight in patients with HIV infection. AIDS 6 (1):
127, 1992. [PUBMED Abstract] Gorter R, Seefried M, Volberding P
http://www.ncbi.nlm.nih.gov/entrez/query.fcgi?cmd=Retrieve&db=Pub
Med&list_uids=1311935&dopt=Abstract

Drugs of Abuse June 15, 2017
https://www.dea.gov/sites/default/files/2018-06/drug_of_abuse.pdf

Drug Enforcement Agency (2013). Phencyclidine. Drug Enforcement
Administration Office of Diversion Control Drug & Chemical

Evaluation Section.

http://www.deadiversion.usdoj.gov/drug_chem_info/pcp.pdf

Effect of cannabinoids on lithium-induced vomiting in the Suncus murinus (house musk shrew). Psychopharmacology (Berl) 171 (2): 156-61, 2004. Parker LA, Kwiatkowska M, Burton P, et al.:
[PUBMED Abstract]

Endocannabinoid modulation of cortical up-states and NREM sleep. PLoS One 9 (2): e88672, 2014. Pava MJ, den Hartog CR, Blanco-Centurion C, et al.:
[PUBMED Abstract]

Endocannabinoid system as an emerging target of pharmacotherapy. Pharmacol Rev 58 (3): 389-462, 2006. Pacher P, Bátkai S, Kunos G:
[PUBMED Abstract]

Endocannabinoids and food intake: newborn suckling and appetite regulation in adulthood. Exp Biol Med (Maywood) 230 (4): 225-34, 2005. Fride E, Bregman T, Kirkham TC:
[PUBMED Abstract]

Endocannabinoids, feeding and suckling--from our perspective. Int J Obes (Lond) 30 (Suppl 1): S24-8, 2006. Mechoulam R, Berry EM, Avraham Y, et al.:
[PUBMED Abstract]

Endogenous cannabinoid system protects against colonic inflammation.

J Clin Invest 113 (8): 1202-9, 2004. Massa F, Marsicano G, Hermann H, et al.:
[PUBMED Abstract]

England, D. (n.d.) PCP Possession and Penalties.
Criminal Defense Lawyer. NOLO
http://www.criminaldefenselawyer.com/resources/pcp-possession-and-penalties.htm

Entopeduncular nucleus endocannabinoid system modulates sleep-waking cycle and mood in rats. Pharmacol Biochem Behav 107: 29-35, 2013. Méndez-Díaz M, Caynas-Rojas S, Arteaga Santacruz V, et al.:
[PUBMED Abstract]

Evaluation of trends in marijuana toxicosis in dogs living in a state with legalized medical marijuana: 125 dogs (2005-2010). Meola SD, Tearney CC, Haas SA, Hackett TB, Mazzaferro EM. J Vet Emerg Crit Care (San Antonio). 2012 Dec;22(6):690-6. doi: 10.1111/j.1476-4431.2012.00818.x.
https://www.ncbi.nlm.nih.gov/pubmed/23216842

Exhaustive List Of Everyone Who's Died Of A Marijuana Overdose By Nick Wing
https://www.huffingtonpost.com/entry/marijuana-lethal-dose_us_58f4ec07e4b0b9e9848d6297

Field Drug Testing: How to Confront False Positives with Expert Testing by Anjelica Cappellino - September 7, 2016 https://www.theexpertinstitute.com/field-drug-testing-how-to-confront-false-positives-with-expert-testing/

First-pass elimination. Basic concepts and clinical consequences. Pond SM, Tozer TN. Clin Pharmacokinet. 1984 Jan-Feb;9(1):1-25. https://www.ncbi.nlm.nih.gov/pubmed/6362950

Florida Man Awarded $37,500 After Cops Mistake Glazed Doughnut Crumbs For Meth October 16, 2017 5:58 PM ET https://www.npr.org/sections/thetwo-way/2017/10/16/558147669/florida-man-awarded-37-500-after-cops-mistake-glazed-doughnut-crumbs-for-meth

Gut Check: Does CBD change to THC in the stomach? https://www.projectcbd.org/gut-check-does-cbd-change-the-stomach

'Helpless': The only treatment for their baby's epileptic seizures was illegal "Every time she has a seizure," said her dad, his voice catching, "to me it's like watching part of her life slip away." - by Rich McHugh / Apr.20.2018 https://www.nbcnews.com/health/kids-health/helpless-only-treatment-their-baby-s-epileptic-seizures-was-illegal-n867626

How long does marijuana stay in your system? How THC blood tests work, and what you should know https://mic.com/articles/168783/how-long-does-marijuana-stay-in-your-system-how-the-blood-tests-work-and-what-you-should-know#.urmND2CqF

Inhibition of colon carcinogenesis by a standardized Cannabis sativa extract with high content of cannabidiol. Phytomedicine 21 (5): 631-9, 2014. Romano B, Borrelli F, Pagano E, et al.:
[PUBMED Abstract]

Inhibition of glioma growth in vivo by selective activation of the CB(2) cannabinoid receptor. Cancer Res 61 (15): 5784-9, 2001. Sánchez C, de Ceballos ML, Gomez del Pulgar T, et al.:
[PUBMED Abstract]

Inhibition of skin tumor growth and angiogenesis in vivo by activation of cannabinoid receptors. J Clin Invest 111 (1): 43-50, 2003. Casanova ML, Blázquez C, Martínez-Palacio J, et al.:
[PUBMED Abstract]

Inhibition of tumor angiogenesis by cannabinoids. FASEB J 17 (3): 529-31, 2003. Blázquez C, Casanova ML, Planas A, et al.:
[PUBMED Abstract]

Inside big pharma's fight to block recreational marijuana
https://www.theguardian.com/sustainable-business/2016/oct/22/recreational-marijuana-legalization-big-business

International Union of Basic and Clinical Pharmacology. LXXIX. Cannabinoid receptors and their ligands: beyond CB_1 and CB_2. Pharmacol Rev 62 (4): 588-631, 2010. [PUBMED Abstract] Pertwee RG, Howlett AC, Abood ME, et al.:

http://www.ncbi.nlm.nih.gov/entrez/query.fcgi?cmd=Retrieve&db=Pub
Med&list_uids=21079038&dopt=Abstract

Involvement of 5HT1A receptors in the anxiolytic-like effects of
cannabidiol injected into the dorsolateral periaqueductal gray of rats.
Psychopharmacology (Berl) 199 (2): 223-30, 2008. Campos AC,
Guimarães FS:
[PUBMED Abstract]

Is CBD Legal? Can CBD Possession Land You in Legal Trouble?
https://theuniversalplant.com/cbd-legal-can-cbd-possession-land-legal-
trouble/

Isolation and structure of a brain constituent that binds to the
cannabinoid receptor. Science 258 (5090): 1946-9, 1992. [PUBMED
Abstract] Devane WA, Hanus L, Breuer A, et al.:
http://www.ncbi.nlm.nih.gov/entrez/query.fcgi?cmd=Retrieve&db=Pub
Med&list_uids=21079038&dopt=Abstract

Lying Drug Tests Incriminate Innocent People
https://www.forbes.com/sites/jacobsullum/2016/07/14/lying-drug-tests-
incriminate-innocent-people/#6a0fa74b3247

Marihuana, The First Twelve Thousand Years. New York: Plenum
Press, 1980. Abel EL
http://www.druglibrary.org/Schaffer/hemp/history/first12000/abel.htm

Marijuana and Medicine: Assessing the Science Base. Washington, DC:

National Academy Press, 1999. Joy JE, Watson SJ, Benson JA, eds.
https://www.nap.edu/read/6376/chapter/1

Marijuana As Medicine? The Science Beyond the Controversy.
Washington, DC: National Academy Press, 2001. Mack A, Joy J
https://www.nap.edu/read/9586/chapter/1

Marijuana Businessman Denied Life Insurance Mutual of Omaha says
pot business employees aren't welcome.
https://www.usnews.com/news/articles/2016-06-23/marijuana-
businessman-denied-life-insurance

Marijuana Is Now Legal In Canada -- Here's Why The U.S. Will Not Be
Far Behind
https://www.forbes.com/sites/jordanwaldrep/2018/06/27/marijuana-is-
now-legal-in-canada-why-the-u-s-will-not-be-far-behind/#47a4ffabbe56

Mast cells express a peripheral cannabinoid receptor with differential
sensitivity to anandamide and palmitoylethanolamide. Proc Natl Acad
Sci U S A 92 (8): 3376-80, 1995. Facci L, Dal Toso R, Romanello S, et
al.:
[PUBMED Abstract]

Medscape.
http://emedicine.medscape.com/article/1010821-medication

Money, Not Morals, Drives Marijuana Prohibition Movement By
Kendall Bentsen August 5, 2014

https://www.opensecrets.org/news/2014/08/money-not-morals-drives-marijuana-prohibition-movement/

More dogs being poisoned by marijuana, vets say, Animal poison control centers report a 'significant increase in the number of calls' related to pets and marijuana by Meghan Holohan / Jul.08.2018 https://www.nbcnews.com/health/health-news/more-dogs-being-poisoned-marijuana-vets-say-n889451

Narconon News (2009).
The History of Drug Abuse and Addiction in America part 6 PCP Retrieved
http://news.narconon.org/history-drug-addiction-pcp-america/http://news.narconon.org/history-drug-addiction-pcp-america/

National Drug Intelligence Center (2013).
PCP Fast Facts. Retrieved
http://www.justice.gov/archive/ndic/pubs4/4440/http://www.justice.gov/archive/ndic/pubs4/4440/

National Toxicology Program: NTP toxicology and carcinogenesis studies of 1-trans-delta(9)-tetrahydrocannabinol (CAS No. 1972-08-3) in F344 rats and B6C3F1 mice (gavage studies). Natl Toxicol Program Tech Rep Ser 446 (): 1-317, 1996.
 [PUBMED Abstract]

Neuro Endocrinol Lett. 2008 Apr;29(2):192-200.
Clinical endocannabinoid deficiency (CECD): can this concept explain

therapeutic benefits of cannabis in migraine, fibromyalgia, irritable bowel syndrome and other treatment-resistant conditions? Russo EB1. https://www.ncbi.nlm.nih.gov/pubmed/18404144

Ninth Circuit Court of Appeals issued a unanimous decision in favor of the HIA February 6, 2004 http://www.votehemp.com/PDF/HIAvDEA_9th_final_decision.pdf

No, CBD Is Not 'Legal In All 50 States' https://www.forbes.com/sites/monazhang/2018/04/05/no-cbd-is-not-legal-in-all-50-states/#d4dad2f762c1

Overdose Death Rates https://www.drugabuse.gov/related-topics/trends-statistics/overdose-death-rates

Pain modulation by release of the endogenous cannabinoid anandamide. Proc Natl Acad Sci U S A 96 (21): 12198-203, 1999. Walker JM, Huang SM, Strangman NM, et al.:
[PUBMED Abstract]

Pathways mediating the effects of cannabidiol on the reduction of breast cancer cell proliferation, invasion, and metastasis. Breast Cancer Res Treat 129 (1): 37-47, 2011. McAllister SD, Murase R, Christian RT, et al.:
[PUBMED Abstract]

Phencyclidine (PCP). (2013, October 29). Retrieved September 9, 2015, from

http://www.cesar.umd.edu/cesar/drugs/pcp.asp

Phytochemical and genetic analyses of ancient cannabis from Central Asia. J Exp Bot 59 (15): 4171-82, 2008. [PUBMED Abstract] Russo EB, Jiang HE, Li X, et al.
http://www.ncbi.nlm.nih.gov/entrez/query.fcgi?cmd=Retrieve&db=Pub Med&list_uids=19036842&dopt=Abstract

PNAS published ahead of print October 5, 2015 A runner's high depends on cannabinoid receptors in mice; Johannes Fuss, Jörg Steinle, Laura Bindila, Matthias K. Auer, Hartmut Kirchherr, Beat Lutz, and Peter Gass
https://doi.org/10.1073/pnas.1514996112

Pot in the workplace: Oregon is No. 1 for positive drug tests
https://www.oregonlive.com/trending/2018/09/pot_in_the_workplace_or egon_ha.html?utm_medium=social&utm_source=facebook&utm_camp aign=theoregonian_sf

Prescription Opioid Data
https://www.cdc.gov/drugoverdose/data/prescribing.html

President Donald J. Trump to Sign Right to Try Legislation
https://www.whitehouse.gov/briefings-statements/president-donald-j-trump-sign-right-try-legislation-fulfilling-promise-made-expand-healthcare-options-terminal-americans/

Professionals Insuring Professionals Attorney Malpractice—Coverage
for Marijuana Practice Up in Smoke?
https://www.l2insuranceagency.com/blog/attorney-malpracticecoverage-
for-marijuana-practice-up-in-smoke.aspx

Prog Neurobiol. 1996 Mar-Apr;48(4-5):275-305.
Cannabinoid receptor genes. Onaivi ES, Chakrabarti A, Chaudhuri G.
https://www.ncbi.nlm.nih.gov/pubmed/8804112

Prog Neurobiol. 2002 Apr;66(5):307-44.
Endocannabinoids and cannabinoid receptor genetics.
Onaivi ES1, Leonard CM, Ishiguro H, Zhang PW, Lin Z, Akinshola BE,
Uhl GR.
https://www.ncbi.nlm.nih.gov/pubmed/12015198

Prostaglandins Leukot Essent Fatty Acids. 2002 Feb-Mar;66(2-3):377-
91. Anandamide receptors. Di Marzo V1, De Petrocellis L, Fezza F,
Ligresti A, Bisogno T.
https://www.ncbi.nlm.nih.gov/pubmed/12052051

Review of the neurological benefits of phytocannabinoids. Maroon J,
Bost J.
Surg Neurol Int. 2018 Apr 26;9:91. doi: 10.4103/sni.sni_45_18.
eCollection 2018.
https://www.ncbi.nlm.nih.gov/pubmed/29770251

S.2667 - Hemp Farming Act of 2018 - 115th Congress (2017-2018)
https://www.congress.gov/bill/115th-congress/senate-bill/2667

Rhode Island gubernatorial, attorney general candidates arrested with 48 pounds of marijuana: police
https://www.foxnews.com/us/rhode-island-gubernatorial-attorney-general-candidates-arrested-with-48-pounds-of-marijuana-police

Schedule of Controlled Substances: Maintaining Marijuana in Schedule...
https://www.deadiversion.usdoj.gov/schedules/marijuana/Maintaining%20Marijuana%20in%20Schedule%201%20of%20the%20Controlled%20Substances%20Act.pdf#search=cbd

Schizophr Res. 2011 Aug;130(1-3):216-21. doi: 10.1016/j.schres.2011.04.017. Epub 2011 May 17. Cannabis with high cannabidiol content is associated with fewer psychotic experiences. Schubart CD1, Sommer IE, van Gastel WA, Goetgebuer RL, Kahn RS, Boks MP.
https://www.ncbi.nlm.nih.gov/pubmed/21592732

Seventeen States Are Flat-Out Ignoring Federal Hemp Laws and Markets Are Thriving
https://fee.org/articles/seventeen-states-are-flat-out-ignoring-federal-hemp-laws-and-markets-are-thriving/

Spain study confirms cannabis oil cures cancer without side effects
http://www.principesactifs.org/spain-study-confirms-cannabis-oil-cures-cancer-without-side-effects/

Structure of cannabidiol: a product isolated from the marihuana extract of Minnesota wild hemp. J Am Chem Soc 62 (1): 196-200, 1940. Adams R, Hunt M, Clark JH:
http://pubs.acs.org/doi/abs/10.1021/ja01858a058

Substance Abuse and Mental Health Services Administration, Center for Behavioral Health Statistics and Quality. (2013).
The DAWN Report: Emergency Department Visits Involving Phencyclidine (PCP). Rockville, MD.
http://www.samhsa.gov/data/sites/default/files/DAWN143/DAWN143/sr143-emergency-phencyclidine-2013.htm

Summary of Decision In *Hemp Industries Ass'n v. Drug Enforcement Admin.*, 333 F.3d 1082 (9th Cir. 2003)
https://web.archive.org/web/20130719092818/http://www.nationalaglawcenter.org/assets/cases/hemp.html

Synergy and phytocannabinoid-terpenoid entourage effects. Br J Pharmacol. 2011;163(7):1344-64.
https://www.ncbi.nlm.nih.gov/pmc/articles/PMC3165946/pdf/bph0163-1344.pdf

Systematic review of the literature on clinical and experimental trials on the antitumor effects of cannabinoids in gliomas. J Neurooncol 116 (1): 11-24, 2014. Rocha FC, Dos Santos Júnior JG, Stefano SC, et al.:
[PUBMED Abstract]

Targeting CB2 cannabinoid receptors as a novel therapy to treat

malignant lymphoblastic disease. Blood 100 (2): 627-34, 2002.
McKallip RJ, Lombard C, Fisher M, et al.:
[PUBMED Abstract]

Tetrahydrocannabinol pharmacokinetics; new synthetic cannabinoids;
road safety and cannabis. [Article in French] Goullé JP, Guerbet M. Bull
Acad Natl Med. 2014 Mar;198(3):541-56; discussion 556-7.
http://europepmc.org/abstract/med/26427296

The Biggest Stoners in Sports (Rolling Stone)
https://www.rollingstone.com/culture/culture-lists/the-biggest-stoners-
in-sports-10982/

The endocannabinoid system as an emerging target of pharmacotherapy.
Pharmacol Rev 58 (3): 389-462, 2006. Pacher P, Bátkai S, Kunos G:
[PUBMED Abstract]
http://www.ncbi.nlm.nih.gov/entrez/query.fcgi?cmd=Retrieve&db=Pub
Med&list_uids=16968947&dopt=Abstract

The First Medicinal Cannabis Kitchen of Its Kind in the Country Will
Debut in Arizona on Friday, Oct. 5
https://www.businesswire.com/news/home/20180912005293/en/Medici
nal-Cannabis-Kitchen-Kind-Country-Debut-Arizona

The Health Effects of Cannabis and Cannabinoids: The Current State of
Evidence and Recommendations for Research. Washington, DC: The
National Academies Press, 2017. National Academies of Sciences,
Engineering, and Medicine

The Marihuana Tax Act of 1937: Taxation of Marihuana. Washington,
DC: House of Representatives, Committee on Ways and Means, 1937.
Schaffer Library of Drug Policy
http://www.druglibrary.org/schaffer/hemp/taxact/woodward.htm

The neurobiology of cannabinoid analgesia. Life Sci 65 (6-7): 665-73,
1999. Walker JM, Hohmann AG, Martin WJ, et al.:
[PUBMED Abstract]

The therapeutic potential of cannabis. Lancet Neurol 2 (5): 291-8, 2003.
Baker D, Pryce G, Giovannoni G, et al.:
[PUBMED Abstract]

Towards the use of cannabinoids as antitumour agents. Nat Rev Cancer
12 (6): 436-44, 2012. Velasco G, Sánchez C, Guzmán M:
[PUBMED Abstract]

Triggering of the TRPV2 channel by cannabidiol sensitizes glioblastoma
cells to cytotoxic chemotherapeutic agents. Carcinogenesis 34 (1): 48-
57, 2013. Nabissi M, Morelli MB, Santoni M, et al.:
[PUBMED Abstract]

U.S. Code › Title 7 › Chapter 88 › Subchapter VII › § 5940
7 U.S. Code § 5940 - Legitimacy of industrial hemp research
https://www.law.cornell.edu/uscode/text/7/5940

Ultimate Guide to Marijuana Use and Insurance 04/19/2017

https://www.huffingtonpost.com/entry/ultimate-guide-to-marijuana-use-and-insurance_us_58f7b9ece4b0c892a4fb74d4

Update on the endocannabinoid system as an anticancer target. Expert Opin Ther Targets 15 (3): 297-308, 2011. Malfitano AM, Ciaglia E, Gangemi G, et al.:
[PUBMED Abstract]

VA and Marijuana – What Veterans need to know
https://www.publichealth.va.gov/marijuana.asp

VA Clears The Air On Doctors Talking To Veterans About Marijuana Use
https://www.npr.org/sections/health-shots/2018/01/09/576577596/va-clears-the-air-on-doctors-talking-to-veterans-about-marijuana-use

Visit Americans for Safe Access to see the specific cannabis laws by state.
https://www.safeaccessnow.org/state_and_federal_law

Warning Letters and Test Results for Cannabidiol-Related Products
https://www.fda.gov/newsevents/publichealthfocus/ucm484109.htm

What is Marijuana really worth?
http://www.priceofweed.com/

Who's Really Fighting Legal Weed - The fight against legal marijuana is about big money, not public health. By Ben Cohen, Contributor   Dec.

8, 2014, at 8:00 a.m.
https://www.usnews.com/opinion/articles/2014/12/08/pot-legalization-opponents-aim-to-protect-their-bottom-line

WikiLeaks Emails Expose Alcohol Industry's Paid Campaign to Stifle Pot Legalization By Matt Agorist - August 8, 2016
https://thefreethoughtproject.com/wikileaks-marijuana-alcohol-lobby/

WikiLeaks Proves the Alcohol Industry Is Working Against Marijuana by Mike Adams | NEWS | Aug 2, 2016
https://merryjane.com/news/wikileaks-proves-the-alcohol-industry-is-working-against-marijuana

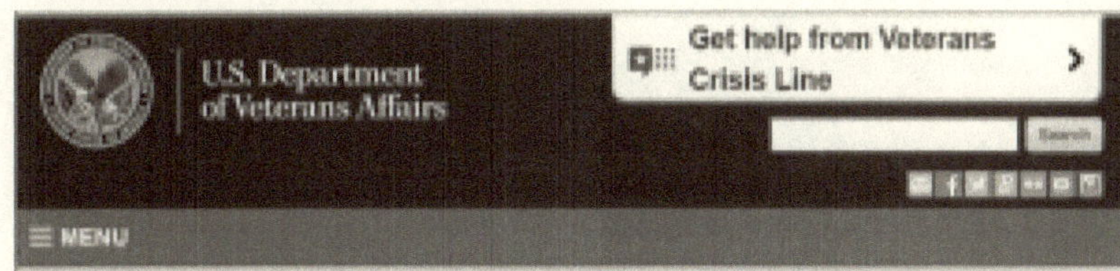

VA » Health Care » Public Health » VA and Marijuana – What Veterans need to know

Public Health

VA and Marijuana – What Veterans need to know

Several states in the U.S. have approved the use of marijuana for medical and/or recreational use. Veterans should know that federal law classifies marijuana – including all derivative products - as a Schedule One controlled substance. This makes it illegal in the eyes of the federal government.

The U.S. Department of Veterans Affairs is required to follow all federal laws including those regarding marijuana. As long as the Food and Drug Administration classifies marijuana as Schedule One VA health care providers may not recommend it or assist Veterans to obtain it.

Veteran participation in state marijuana programs does not affect eligibility for VA care and services. VA providers can and do discuss marijuana use with Veterans as part of comprehensive care planning, and adjust treatment plans as necessary.

Some things Veteran need to know about marijuana and the VA:

- Veterans will not be denied VA benefits because of marijuana use.
- Veterans are encouraged to discuss marijuana use with their VA providers.

- VA health care providers will record marijuana use in the Veteran's VA medical record in order to have the information available in treatment planning. As with all clinical information, this is part of the confidential medical record and protected under patient privacy and confidentiality laws and regulations.
- VA clinicians may not recommend medical marijuana.
- VA clinicians may only prescribe medications that have been approved by the FDA for medical use. At present most products containing Tetrahydrocannabinol (THC), Cannabidiol (CBD), or other cannabinoids are not approved for this purpose.
- VA clinicians may not complete paperwork/forms required for Veteran patients to participate in state-approved marijuana programs.
- VA pharmacies may not fill prescriptions for medical marijuana.
- VA will not pay for medical marijuana prescriptions from any source.
- VA scientists may conduct research on marijuana benefits and risks, and potential for abuse, under regulatory approval. Please address questions related to research to: VHABLRD-CSRD@va.gov
- The use or possession of marijuana is prohibited at all VA medical centers, locations and grounds. When you are on VA grounds it is federal law that is in force, not the laws of the state.
- Veterans who are VA employees are subject to drug testing under the terms of employment.

View the full directive "Access to VHA Clinical Programs for Veterans Participating in State-Approved Marijuana Programs (73 KB, PDF)." (VHA Directive 1315)

If you have questions regarding this policy please contact: population.health@va.gov

Emails sent to this address are not secure. Please do not include personal data. To send a secure email, use VA's Ask a Question - IRIS (a secure website contracted to VA).

Keywords: cannabinoids, terpenoids, essential oils, THC, CBD, CBG, CBA, CBN, limonene, pinene, linalool, caryophyllene, phytotherapy, Biology, Medicine, Treatment

Page Intentionally Left Blank for Your Own Notes:

About The Author

Personally, I have been active in the Health Industry, for people and animals, primarily dealing with joints and digestion, with some a small amount of time regarding critical care meals, reproduction supplements, and general health primarily for MD's Choice, Inc. since 1995.

I was armed with a decent brain, some awesome mentors, and a meniscal degree in Physical Sciences from the 80's. I'd like to believe I have a pile of common sense, some rational logic, and an ethical desire to find some truth more often than not. Over the years, I have edited thousands of pages for doctors I've been working with. They insisted that I learn about health and nutrition, and grilled me… correcting, and teaching me over the years, as I selected and edited the content and maintained dozens of health related websites, nearly 100 product labels, marketing materials and advertisements over the last twenty plus years.

Ultimately, in the Health Industry, I am just a well-trained parrot, with an understanding of my own limitations, and foundation of experience.

Growing up I heard people joke about 'those people' that were a 'jack of all trades, but a master of NONE.' I quickly realized I did not want to be like that. However, I also didn't really want to 'put all my eggs in one basket' as many in the timber industry had done in my small Southern Oregon hometown, which lost everything, their homes, retirement, and entire life savings, over a spotted owl controversy that was really never a problem (because of the logging or timber industry).

I tried to focus on a few topics, learn all I could about them, master those that were important to me and my goals. I knew, with the topics I selected, no matter how much I learned, there would always be more to learn. New stuff, and skills to refine, because of the constant changes and technical evolution in those fields over time. Tough to get bored with things that are never stagnate. Perfect, for me.

The majority of my life has been focused on helping solve problems, making money, computers, cameras, marketing, health, nutrition, scuba diving, learning, doing, and then helping educate others most of the nearly sixty years of my life.

BUSINESS VENTURES & JOBS:

MD's Choice, Inc. – 1995 to present - President and Co-founder, introduce company and products to the world, through both active and passive marketing, and fact-based advertising, with the goal of education and quality solutions. My focus is on making things presentable to the public, both aesthetically and in a fashion any normal person can understand. I deal with the product labeling, marketing material designs, advertising, trade shows, and web sites. I stumbled across the right questions, which led to one of our patented multi-species repro products.

TerryMercer.com – 2001 to present – Sponsored Professional Cameraman – Freelance Writer, mostly on topics of photography, and camera use. Primarily Sports Action, Nature, and Music Concerts (Events).

PBG – June 1991-June 2006, restated 2012 to present – for some web design projects. Owner-Operator-Computer Hardware & Software - focused on small business & education; small business consulting, custom web development, technical support reduction, and custom software design and testing. (Started as a partnership, between Dynamic Solutions and another Southern Oregon company, which I later bought out my partner in 1993).

TackStore Info & Key Marketing Solutions.org – 2004 to 2012 – Co-founder, with Ralph D' Agosta (America's Areas) – My responsibilities were-data base acquisition and management, both mailer and website design and management, and monthly articles. TackStoreInfo.com – was a viable resource for the 36,000 Wholesale Buyers in the Equine Industry, promoting products, information to help small businesses compete better, and dealing with some of the industry changes and politics. It was a quarterly direct mailer, and website with monthly articles.

Freelance Writing – mostly for a variety of computer related (hardware & software) trade & consumer magazines (CD Rom Today, Replication News, Software Tomorrow, Shareware Magazine, and other industry magazines). As well as some newspaper articles and contributions, and 'ratings' (movies and products). Step-by-step instructions for HOW TO use, do, fix, repair, upgrade, clean or deal with certain specific items. Generally, jobs, tools, or computerized equipment or software... regarding computer peripherals, scuba diving, cameras (photography), certain topics on health and nutrition, and raising kids.

Micromedia, Inc. – April 1991-August 1998 – President (title) - Contract Negotiation and 'making vapor real' (ie, sourcing, testing, and licensing software programs, creating product, project development, organization of data to CD mastering, and management of projects). I was the chief nerd until things started happening I didn't like... so I walked away late summer 98, deciding to put more effort into helping build MD's Choice.

Southern Oregon State College (SOSC) – 1991-1993 – Instructor: - Taught Computer courses - hardware (build & repair) and software (OS & business applications, Word, Excel, Publisher, QuickBooks, etc.). I developed the curriculum & syllabus from scratch, because at that time mostly only programming courses had predefined curriculum. Each semester was tailored to the individuals in the classes, and the goals of the majority - a) continuing education, b) work study, c) vocational. I held a vote as the start of each class, with a majority rule - why they were there and what they wanted to learn.

In 1993, my private consulting business, technical support reduction, web design, and teaching were all put on the proverbial back burner when our CD-ROM development and software design enhancements companies finally took off. I did not have the time for the other projects, so I paid off any debt, and shelved all I could (put in notice where necessary, and helped my clients find a replacement).

Structured teaching was fun, interesting, and frankly gave me an appreciation of how much teachers, instructors, and professors work outside of the class room - creating course work, curriculum, syllabuses, reading each of the student's papers and grading tests. WOW... much more than I had previously imagined.

Dynamic Solutions – February 1989 - September 1992 – President (title)-Custom Computer Hardware - both high end desk tops, lunch boxes, and note books... with appropriate software installed, tested, and customer's trained. Built customer computers for thousands of businesses in the USA, as well as specialty computers for Liton Industries, and Met One Technologies. (It was bought out, and merged with PBG).

PSI Research, Inc.(Oasis Press) -1988 - 1995-VP of Information Technology. I dealt with the hardware & software decisions - both for internal use & maintenance & management, as well as the software we developed for resale in the business market. I became a consultant to the company in 1994, continuing to supply their computer needs, off-site technical support, and trained my replacements, Ken Clever and Ted

Weiss. Thanks to Emmet Ramey, who helped me officially start Dynamic Solutions. I helped as needed, as my business ventures grew.

US. Air Force – 1978 - Honorable Medical Discharge

Favorite Topics & Activities – Health and Nutrition, Computers, Cameras, Marketing, Business, Family, Scuba Diving, U.S. Constitution, Aquariums, Bald Eagles, Beaches, Outdoors, Biking, Boating, Bowling, Create Things, Creativity, Cycling, Eight ball, Entrepreneurialism, Extreme Sports, Fiction writing, Freelance Writing, Friends, Horseback Riding, Inventing, Kayaking, Martial arts, Nature, Nine-ball, Outdoor activities, Philosophy, Photography, Poetry Writing, Politics, Positive Thinking, Psychology, Quading, Research, RVing, Science, Sightseeing, Snowmobiling, Sociology, Spearfishing, Swimming, Technology, Texas Holdem, Thinking, Traveling, Video games, Weight Lifting, White Water, Wildlife, Writing Books, Zip lining, , and many other things,

Favorite Books - Laws of Power, Atlas Shrugged, Brave New World, Eat Love Pray, Fahrenheit 451, Veterinary Handbook, How to Talk to a Liberal, Illusions, Laws of Karma, Love and Survival, Love by Leo Buscaglia, Napoleon Hill -Think and Grow Rich, Pay It Forward, Self-help, Sun Tzu The Art of War, The Art of Happiness, The Bridge Across Forever, A Lovestory, Johnathon Livingston Seagull, The Count of Monte Cristo, The Giver, The Last Lecture (book), The Last Lecture Randy Pausch, The Notebook, The Power of Now, The Secret, Weapons of Mass Distortion, Crime fiction,

Some Personal Experience:

I grew up in S. Oregon N. California... that geographical area was the pot capital of the world in the 60's and 70's. Frankly, I think there are two 'types' of people that generally used marijuana back in the 60's & 70's.

-	Those that just wanted the high, the escape, the party... and
-	those that were hyper active and needed the calm

Frankly, neither really cared what other's thought, during those years, and might not have let others know they were 'dong it' outside their tight group of friends.

I've known Eagle Scouts that smoked weed on a regular basis, as well as people that went on to get PhD's, and even build multi-million dollar businesses; that chose pot over alcohol or abstinence.

WHEN those I've known over the years decided to 'indulge,' the vast majority were nice and friendly people, more 'laid back' and more of the stereo-typical 'peace and love to everybody' sort of actions (and attitude). **Many would literally give you the shirt off their back, even if they might need it** (though those willing to go to that extreme were rare, most only if it didn't short them).

Personally, I'd rather see cannabis legalized over alcohol, as there are far fewer instances of violence, blackouts, aggressive anger issues, auto-accidents, toxic build up, or overdose impact than either alcohol or most pain relievers. Cannabis based products are safer than alcohol, healthier than cigarettes, and often times sincerely have medical benefits that have been scientifically supported in study results.

But that's my experience, bias, and knowledge on the topic. Because it is against the law, I haven't indulged... because I have multiple business ventures, and occasional FDA inspections already (for the Nutritional Business), I likely wouldn't... unless there was a specific medical reason (like I had a type of cancer it would likely help).

And then, I would bother to a) listen to my doctor(s), and b) make sure I was using the RIGHT TYPE, with the correct foundational nutrients... which are not just CBD, and usually also a ratio of THC when it comes to dealing with things like Cancer. LOOK AT QUALITY ABSTRACTS and real science. Talk to real doctors, question real researchers... and please do not try to purchase hope or promises from TV commercials or celebrities!

THE
SORCERER'S GUIDE
TO THE

SOUL OF
ANESIDORA

L. SCOTT CLARK

ISBN: 978-1-954814-06-6 (Paperback)
ISBN: 978-1-954814-09-7 (Hardcover)
ISBN: 978-1-954814-07-3 (EBook)
ISBN: 978-1-954814-08-0 (Audiobook)
Library of Congress Control Number: 2021921871

First Edition 2021

Credits:
Book Cover and Formatting by Miblart — www.miblart.com
Editing by Elite Editing — https://eliteediting.com

Obsidian Wolf Publishing
www.obsidianwolfpub.com
PO Box 1086
Salem, UT 84653